T0235065

Paternal Postnatal Psychiatric Illnesses

Shaila Kulkarni Misri

Paternal Postnatal Psychiatric Illnesses

A Clinical Case Book

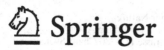
Springer

Shaila Kulkarni Misri
University of British Columbia
Vancouver, BC, Canada

ISBN 978-3-319-68248-8   ISBN 978-3-319-68249-5   (eBook)
https://doi.org/10.1007/978-3-319-68249-5

Library of Congress Control Number: 2017957711

Printed on acid-free paper

This Springer imprint is published by Springer Nature
The registered company is Springer International Publishing AG
The registered company address is: Gewerbestrasse 11, 6330 Cham, Switzerland

This book is written in the memory of my mother who advocated for destigmatizing depression and anxiety. She inspired me to follow a career in medicine.

I thank Nicholas, my son and now a fellow psychiatrist, for his steadfast support and reassurance. I am appreciative of Nathaniel and Tiffany, my son and daughter-in-law, for their encouragement.

Most of all, I remain grateful to Bushan, my husband, for his unconditional and tireless support through my long journey as a psychiatrist. His unwavering faith in my work makes me propel forward.

Preface

This book is long overdue. Despite the current advances in the area of perinatal mental health, emotional sufferings of a new dad appear to have been hidden in plain sight. A variety of reasons account for this reality. While stigma and embarrassment associated with disclosing psychological struggles after childbirth is a significant factor, lack of awareness on the part of health-care providers may explain this gap. Typically, joy, excitement and contentment are expected of a man when he embarks on the journey of fatherhood. Revealing angst, fear and sorrow associated with the birth of his newborn can be interpreted as a sign of weakness. As a result, psychiatric disorders in new fathers frequently go undiagnosed and untreated. Suffering in silence is the rule for these dads. Their emotional upheaval and anguish tends to manifest in a variety of pathological ways which include mood and anxiety problems, substance use, marital dissatisfaction and attachment issues with the baby, to name a few. Dads' psychological impairment has detrimental effect on the dynamics of the new family, both in the short term and in the long term.

I have attempted to increase awareness of this as yet under-researched area that should be on the radar of clinicians who treat mental health issues during child-bearing age, both in females and in males. It is our responsibility to make the new dad feel at ease when he decides to share symptoms of panic attacks while visiting his 2-day infant in the hospital; we want to be compassionate to the dad who is consumed with irrational worry of baby's safety; we do not want to be in judgement of the father who starts to drink excessively because of the added responsibility of his baby; we have to be sensitive to new dads who disclose their sexual misgivings after childbirth. Finally, we must be mindful and alert of a depressed dad with thoughts of suicide.

The book offers up-to-date overview of commonly encountered psychiatric disorders in new dads that are relevant in clinical practice. This volume, I trust, will serve as a resource for a variety of health-care providers such as psychiatrists, psychologists, obstetricians, family doctors, nurses and social workers, midwives and doulas who strive to deliver high-quality care to their perinatal patients. Most importantly, my hope is that this book will encourage new dads to come forward with their concerns, however minuscule, and seek help in a timely manner.

I am indebted to Isabel Sadowski without whom this book would not have been a reality. She spent inordinate amount of time on this book with me every step of the way. Isabel, you are awesome! Contributions of Ashley and Sue Han have been invaluable. Lorraine, I appreciate the flawless transcription. I also want to thank Nadina Persaud, Associate Editor, Springer, who believed that I had something worthwhile to convey to my readership. Lastly, I remain grateful to the partners of my female patients; they taught me to listen to their stories and helped me understand their strife of being a new father.

Vancouver, BC, Canada   Shaila Kulkarni Misri

Contents

Chapter 1
History of Postpartum Psychiatric Disorders: Don't Forget the Dads

Pregnancy and child birth affect both men and women's lives. But, historically, it has always been women's perinatal signs and symptoms that have been focused on by obstetricians and other health-care providers. In the 1930s, however males' emotional difficulties began to be documented. In the twenty-first century, although there appears to be growing interest in the psychological well-being of the new dad, not much attention has been paid to this issue in a scientific manner. As a result, it has not been acknowledged to the extent it deserves. Furthermore, while knowledge with regard to psychiatric illnesses in new mothers has made strides, fathers have been left behind. This has impacted the overall well-being of the family unit. Not providing psychological intervention to a new dad also influences the maternal recovery from mental illness. Maternal postpartum psychiatric disorders are less stigmatized today than they were earlier; however, this cannot be said about paternal psychological illnesses that appear to be equally prevalent but as yet go unnoticed. In this book, I attempt to bring to the attention of my readers the internal turmoil faced by new dads that is often forgotten in the light of the birth of a new baby.

Men undergoing physical changes related to pregnancy in their wife were mentioned by doctors in the form of "couvade syndrome". Couvade syndrome is a psychogenic disorder which affects husbands during their wives' pregnancies or parturition. While there are many different symptoms that are described in

© Springer International Publishing AG 2018

S.K. Misri, *Paternal Postnatal Psychiatric Illnesses*,
https://doi.org/10.1007/978-3-319-68249-5_1

the expectant father, the most striking resemble those from which pregnant women commonly suffer. These include gastrointestinal issues such as appetite change, indigestion, weight gain, diarrhoea or constipation. Occasionally the vomiting and nausea that their pregnant partners suffer from are also mimicked by the suffering husbands. These symptoms that correspond with the wife's pregnancy disappear in the male once their wife gives birth. It is seen in modern psychiatry as an expression of somatized anxiety, identification with the foetus as well as ambivalence about fatherhood in general. In earlier psychodynamic terms, it also indicates a statement of paternity and/or envy of parturition or childbirth. The presentation of different types of symptomatology generally varies between individuals and appears to be multidimensional. It appears that the incidence of couvade syndrome varies from 11% to 65% depending on the cultural context. Essentially, the phenomenon of couvade points to the intimacy of the father to his child by experiencing some of the symptoms that mimic the signs of pregnancy.

The origin of this syndrome lies in the French word "couver" which means to "hatch or sit on". In anthropological and etymological terms, "couver" denotes various rituals for the father during the time of childbirth. For instance, around the time of childbirth, the father goes to bed and behaves as if he was going through delivery pains himself. It could be that the father deals with these feelings of empathy with his wife by experiencing these symptoms himself and/or he could also imitate his wife's symptoms as he feels left out and envious that she is the one who is going through the actual bearing of the child while he is an onlooker. Lastly, it could be one of the ways or mechanisms in which husband reacts to the ambivalent relationship between the couple, where the wife may not be sexually available towards the end of the pregnancy, or may not provide the intimacy that the husband is looking for. This may explain why he expresses his internal conflict in this manner as he may hope that their relationship will be in some way protected as a result. Another way of identifying with a pregnant partner would be to refrain from eating certain foods. This is because the partner is not able to eat certain foods and must stick to a specific diet, especially if she is nauseous. It could also be a way to protect the baby from hostile impulses that the father may have towards it. So, it appears that Couvade syndrome contains certain self-punitive aspects affecting the father. According to some researchers who have taken more in-depth looks into couvade syndrome, it appears that this particular condition can be considered as a somatic equivalent of primitive rituals in recognizing the beginning of fatherhood.

In the modern world, a similar type of psychodynamic prevails and makes its appearance in a different cultural context. In my practice I frequently come across expectant fathers who show nesting behaviours in anticipation of the birth of a newborn; this is generally seen as a positive participation in the face of new parenthood and is generally met with approval, respect and compliments. At other times, I often come across would-be dads who inadvertently gain weight with each trimester of his partner's pregnancy. Generally such men after childbirth will show different physical ways of expressing anxiety when they embark upon the new task of being a dad. Societal expectations for new dads have gone on a dramatic shift, especially in the past 25–30 years. This occurs more so in the western world than many of the other developing countries. Referring to the notion of paternity leave, while this concept is a sign of giving the new dad an equal opportunity to participate in the upbringing of his newborn, biologically speaking, he hasn't had the time to adjust to the experience of perinatal changes. Sociologically, however, the expectation that he would rise to the occasion of being an exceptional, talented and intuitive new dad can place a huge burden for most males. Under these circumstances, expressing feelings of fear, conflict or concerns around this new role could be seen as an embarrassing admission of a new dad's inadequacy. Competitive feelings about mastery over fatherhood are often seen along with the attendant sense of angst they produce.

Masoni and his colleagues conducted an interesting study of 73 couples where women in the last trimester of pregnancy were given a questionnaire, and as a control group, 73 men without pregnant wives or children under 1 year of age were recruited. An emotional involvement connected to pregnancy was reported in 91.78% of the participants. This was expressed either in the forms of sexual habits (87.67%) or fear and anxiety (36.98%) and finally curiosity in about 50%. It appears from the findings of this study that some males about to become fathers possibly experience a change in their behaviour or their thinking as they embark on fatherhood. It appears that the psychological response to being a new father occurs with more frequency than has been recognized. It is generally the mother who receives the attention, whether during pregnancy or in the postpartum period, thereby almost overlooking the significant role of the father. Men also present with complicated responses or reactions to the birth of their children. While many males do respond positively to becoming fathers, others may go through a more difficult journey in order to integrate into their new role. Despite the pleasure and joy experienced by men in becoming new fathers, it is not uncommon for them to experience a variety of psychiatric difficulties when transitioning through this important aspect of their lives.

What is unclear with respect to non-specific psychological changes that an expectant father may go through is whether all of these resolve completely or if residual symptoms of psychiatric conflicts continue to manifest themselves after the birth of the baby. This is because long-term prospective data on these fathers who have gone through the pregnancy is not available. Presently, psychiatric symptomatology in new fathers is seen as having its onset after childbirth, without having much understanding of their conflict and/or ability to come to terms with their new role during the pregnancy. While the female has a chance to prepare herself through the physiological, anatomical and psychological changes of pregnancy for 40 weeks, the envy in the male associated with the inability to experience similar changes may lead, in certain vulnerable individuals, to not accepting the reality of the responsibilities that go with becoming a father. The birth of a child adds a substantial amount of responsibility onto the father, as typically the mother is no longer working and is on maternity leave in the modern world. In reality, this does interrupt the career of the mother, thereby increasing the financial burden on the father. Secondly, it appears that the shift in the marital relationship towards becoming less intimate with one another and more with the child can be another interesting factor that might create a further barrier to sexual and emotional intimacy. Often, the father feels left out while the mother is busy with her child, especially in the first few weeks when nursing is being established. If it is a male child, often fathers may feel envious or jealous of this new male in their partner's life, and in some individuals, this may also bring about gender-related conflicts that were absent or not obvious to him up to that point.

Individuals who have had a difficult or conflictual relationship with their own parents may have difficulty becoming a father, as some of these intense, unresolved feelings from the past may surface and interfere with the relationship with their own children. Unlike the common myth that a baby can bind a marriage, it would appear that the birth of a child in an unsatisfactory union may actually lead to separation or divorce if the conflicts become unbearable for both partners. The unconscious hostility towards the newborn or infant may become an issue for both parents. Therefore, the presence of a newborn markedly changes the dynamics of both parents. However, all of the factors discussed thus far are not unusual in most marriages and/or families. The important predictors that increase an individual's vulnerability with regard to the onset of psychiatric symptoms in the postpartum period remain as yet unclear; however, in this book, an attempt will be made to illustrate some of the complexities that accompany fatherhood beyond what is considered to be "normal". Sometimes it is not easy to delineate between what is normal and what is abnormal. Generally, the passage of time or visits with the family, and especially face-to-face interview with the couple on a regular basis, and collateral information from the mother identifies a partner who is at risk for experiencing psychiatric symptoms. A detailed history and examination to enquire and understand the relationship between the parents, as well as the reaction to fatherhood, are important before a psychiatric label should be placed upon the new father.

The value of recognizing the illness in the father is not to further stigmatize the family, but to establish guidelines for both the parents to be able to parent in an effective way. This will help to prevent the baby from being impacted by the ongoing conflict and emotional upheaval, which in both the short and long term have proven to have adverse impacts on the development of the child. As yet, there is a lack of systematic research on paternal psychiatric disorders that would help clinicians diagnose in a timely manner and provide appropriate interventions. Emotional issues associated with fatherhood are quite common. Earlier studies showed that 2% of patients hospitalized with paranoid psychoses were cases triggered by fatherhood. No single mental illness is specifically associated with fatherhood; a wide range of symptoms and syndromes with functional as well as psychological overlays are encountered. Review papers in available literature from the 1950s to 1960s focused on mild to severe neurotic tendencies and characterological disorders, sexual deviation as well as psychosomatic illnesses and functional psychoses in fathers.

A variety of different authors have attempted to review paternal psychiatric disorders. Zilborg in 1931 discusses the psychodynamic aspects and elaborates on depressive reactions related to parenthood. Thirty patients in his sample were described as having depressive reactions to parenthood, of which two or three experienced a psychotic aspect at the time of the wife's pregnancy. The author's interpretation was that these psychotic depressions had paranoid dimensions to them. In 1951, Freeman and colleagues examined pregnancy as a precipitant of mental illness in fathers. They presented six cases, and one of them was admitted to an inpatient facility. This particular father experienced a paranoid type of psychotic reaction, possibly schizophrenic in nature, associated with his wife's pregnancy. Two other patients admitted were diagnosed with severe bipolar disorder. They exhibited symptoms of rage, some somatic delusions as well as fear of death. The last three experienced depression, anxiety and hypochondriacal fears.

In 1951, Curtis described a cohort of 55 expectant fathers and their corresponding psychiatric symptomatology. He divided the fathers into three groups: those with major psychiatric problems, those with minor psychiatric problems and those without. The two groups with psychiatric problems were referred from a military setting. The most severe group presented with impulsive behaviour disorders, borderline personality issues as well as psychosomatic problems. Most frequently, they had a history of impulsive behaviour, had lower enlisted ranks, were known for their misconduct or were unmarried and were showing open rejection of the baby. Wives had experienced past psychiatric illness and were also presently showing emotional lability. Towne and Afterman, in their 1955 description of psychoses in males related to parenthood, surveyed a large population of a Virginia hospital for schizophrenic patients and those whose breakdowns were triggered by fatherhood. Of the 879 patients diagnosed with schizophrenia, 18 were found to have their symptoms associated with fatherhood. Previously, ten other similar patients were also located from an acute treatment programme in the same hospital. A total of 28 patients were acutely disturbed upon admission, but required less than a month of hospitalization, and improved at the time of discharge. Many of these patients had experienced parental deprivation, with early tumultuous family issues in their own lives.

In 1962, Jarvis presented two patients with characterological reactions to fatherhood and also discussed two other men who showed different compensatory mechanisms after the birth of a child. For instance, one became psychotic, while the other had dependency needs and became involved in an affair and increasingly estranged during his wife's pregnancy, as a result. Another interesting way of coping with childbirth was reported by Hartmann and Nicolay and manifested in the form of sexual deviancies such as voyeurism, exhibitionism and rape. Postpartum psychosis in males is also not a rare phenomenon. Retterstol examined a series of first admissions of male patients with paranoid psychotic reactions in the psychiatric department of a hospital at Oslo University in 1968.

Of the 169 patients that were admitted, fatherhood was an important trigger for reactive psychosis in four. Of these, two became seriously ill right after childbirth. It is interesting to review the historical perspective of the psychiatric symptomatology in males, whether it is in the late trimester of pregnancy or early in the postpartum period. Early literature showed that most of these fathers responded to childbirth by experiencing a delusional state with inpatient hospitalization, as well as reactive depressive symptoms, and, finally, with behavioural disorders such as sexual deviation and/or dysfunctional behaviours when they become new fathers.

This type of presentation in new fathers could reflect the evolution of the paternal role over the past two or three centuries. For instance, fathers are now becoming an integral part of pregnancy as well as the birthing process; it is more common than not for a father to attend prenatal classes, to be present in the birthing room and, finally, to be a "hands-on" father compared to his predecessors only 10 or 20 years ago. This evolution of the role of the expectant father could possibly explain why the response to fatherhood, as far as psychiatric symptoms are concerned, is not as intense as the psychotic reactions that were seen 30 or 40 years ago. It appears that males feel less stigmatized with regard to talking about their "feelings" as there is more acceptance with regard to their transition to parenthood. Paternal leave is offered in several parts of the world now, which legitimizes their struggle with fatherhood, as it does for mothers as well.

I have not come across any psychotic fathers in my practice of over 35 years. This may have largely to do with the type of patients who come to see us at the psychiatric clinic which is attached to a maternity hospital in an urban setting, as well as the demographics of the patients who attend such a clinic. I decided to write this book not to frighten the new moms or dads, but to help the health caregivers so as to not miss identifying those who need intervention. Not much is written about the strife of new dads. Mother is the centre of attention and rightfully so; however, in a modern household, in the absence of the support of extended family, fathers shoulder the complete responsibility of the newborn along-side the mother. They go through the fears, qualms as well as uncertainties related to this new transition. In heterosexual relationships, the difference between fathers and their part-ners is that the woman tends to get care and consideration, while the man is left to fend for himself. The end result is a chronic sense of inadequacy, self-doubt and apprehension. In some vulnerable fathers, this may lead to the manifestation of emotional instability and the eventual appearance of psychi-atric symptomatology.

My goal is to educate clinicians such as physicians, mid-wives, perinatal nurses, doulas, psychologists, counsellors, social workers and many other health-care professionals that are engaged in providing care to the new mother, to not for-get the needs of the fathers. They deserve to be noticed; they must be encouraged to be included and most importantly, not be made to feel embarrassed if deemed to experience signs of mental instability. Although stories of dads in this book are real, I have done my best not to break confidentiality by changing their circumstances as well as the settings. I remain forever grateful to for them giving me the opportunity to be "an insider" and sharing with me their private thoughts and feelings without any reservation. I feel privileged to earn their confidence and trust. This book would not have been a reality without their input.

References

1. Curtis JL. A psychiatric study of fifty-five expectant fathers. U S Armed Forces Med J. 1955;6:937–50.
2. Dawson WR. The custom of couvade. Manchester: Manchester University Press; 1929.
3. Freeman T. Pregnancy as a precipitant of mental illness in men. Brit J Med Psychol. 1951;24:49–54.
4. Hartman AA, Nicolay R. Sexually deviant behavior in expectant fathers. J Abnorm Psychol. 1966;71:232–4.
5. Jarvis W. Some effects of pregnancy and childbirth on men. J Am Psychoanal Assn. 1962;10:689–700.

6. Lacoursiere RB. Fatherhood and mental illness: a review and new material. Psychiatry Q. 1972;46(1):109–24.
7. Masoni S, Maio A, Trimarchi G, et al. The couvade syndrome. J Psychosom Obstet Gynaecol. 1994;15(3):125–31.
8. Retterstol N. Paranoid psychoses associated with impending or newly established fatherhood. Acta Psychiatr Scand. 1968;44:51–61.
9. Towne RD, Afterman J. Psychosis in males related to parenthood. Bull Menn Clin. 1955;19:19–26.
10. Wainwright WH. Fatherhood as a precipitant of mental illness. Am J Psychiatry. 1966;123(1):40–4.
11. Zilboorg C. Depressive reactions related to parenthood. Am J Psychiatry. 1931;87:927–62.

Chapter 2
Paternal Postpartum Depression: A Sad Dad

Dad's Story: Clinical Vignette

John was an only child to his parents who had high expectations for him as he grew up. John came from a fairly privileged family; he went to good schools when young and did very well in university. In keeping with his family's wishes, he went to law school where he graduated with highest distinction. He aspired to follow the footsteps of his father and grandfather who were both eminent lawyers. They were proud to have him carry forward the family legacy.

Growing up, John excelled in almost everything he did. He played sports competitively, did a lot of community work, and joined various overseas volunteer organizations; it was anticipated that he would be very successful. He continued to shine throughout his adulthood outside of his academic prowess by assisting his mother in fundraising organizations and was very compassionate towards female equality and supporting females in the profession of law. When he met Katie during law school, it appeared he had found the perfect partner. Together, they were a young power couple who had a lot of dreams and aspirations for themselves, including the creation of a family.

(continued)

© Springer International Publishing AG 2018
S.K. Misri, *Paternal Postnatal Psychiatric Illnesses*,
https://doi.org/10.1007/978-3-319-68249-5_2

They bought a small condominium close to Katie's parents and started working full time soon after graduating from law school. They made specific choices with regards to a work/life balance by dividing the type of law practice they would pursue. For instance, he decided to join a large, national firm downtown, while Katie decided to pursue a job as in-house counsel with benefits including maternity leave. This choice was made as John was going to be the principal bread-winner of the family, and Katie would be the caretaker, as was the trajectory in his own family.

The pregnancy was planned. Katie was already well over 2 years into her job; she had secured a good, stable position with an environmental law firm and was very happy to become pregnant. All the medical visits were satisfactory and the pregnancy went well. Throughout the pregnancy, the couple attended prenatal classes. This was a pleasant change for John whose father did not participate much in John's life when he was young. His father frequently travelled and was away during John's formative years. John did not want to follow the same pattern of parenting when he became a father himself. This led to him being involved in fatherhood right from the start by going shopping with Katie, painting the nursery and purchasing necessary items for the baby.

Katie had normal labour and vaginal delivery, and it was a perfect case scenario in the labour room, with John helping, as was expected of him. Julie was a full-term baby, healthy at 8 8 lbs.; she brought a lot of joy to her parents. However, within the first 4 weeks of bringing Julie home, Katie began to experience sleepless nights, and worry about the baby, especially around nursing issues. Also, Julie was difficult to soothe, and would cry through the night. Many nights, Katie would be up trying to console the infant, rocking back and forth, or walking around. John was helping around the clock, trying to be supportive. Katie became more anxious, her crying spells increased and her detachment towards Julie became more obvious.

(continued)

He took a few days of leave to support Katie; he could not ask for longer leave as big cases were being handled by the firm and he was primarily responsible for many of the files. Work started to pile up. In the meantime, the situation at home began to deteriorate

Around this point in time, John felt concerned about his baby's welfare and stepped up his parental responsibility. He would be up most nights trying to assist with Julie's feeding schedule, but found it a very frustrating experience. After a few weeks, the baby switched to bottle feeding. Waking up exhausted and tired, John began to get agitated himself. At work, he found that he could not focus and his concentration was impaired. After about 3 or 4 months of decreased productivity at work, his colleague spoke to him politely and shared that there were some concerns about his performance and absenteeism. Not paying much attention to his co-worker's concerns, John continued to accompany Katie to doctors' appointments. Katie, who was diagnosed with postpartum depression, did not like to drive, so she was completely dependent on John for getting to these appointments.

John found that he was becoming increasingly distressed with the passage of time. The lack of emotional access to his wife, who appeared to be more distant and short-fused, was hard for him to cope with. John did not want to talk to his male friends about his plight and started to isolate himself. Gradually, he became introverted. There were no more after-work drinks with his male colleagues, and no more basketball games. He spent his evenings at home with Katie and Julie, waking up dog-tired day after day. John started to experience insomnia; he began to overeat; he found himself going to food for comfort. His overall motivation diminished. His pleasure over any meaningful activities in life decreased significantly. Most of all, he felt alarmed about feeling distant from his little girl, who he had waited so long to

(continued)

have in his life. He felt angry, detached, and suffered from feelings of guilt as a result.

Eventually, these various aspects of fatherhood that were now negatively impacting him as well as his family, came to a head when John was given notice of termination from his firm. He could not, in his wildest dreams, ever imagine that the first few years of his law career would potentially end up in shambles. He had dreams of making partner some day. He dreaded that this opportunity was now taken away from him. He felt extremely demoralized. He had a lot of guilt, and blamed himself that he had let his family down. His mother in the meantime kept asking him whether she could be of help. Katie's mother also offered to spend nights at their place to help with the baby. Both of them were too proud to accept a helping hand from their mothers. Having their mothers involved in childcare was seen by them as a failure in their parenting skills. They were determined to do it themselves; they did not mobilize their social supports and tried to deal with the battle of new parenthood on their own.

John began to feel sad and anxious about the future, which appeared to be bleak. He was desperately looking for answers. He was trying to understand what it was that he was going through and why he dreaded everyday. His negative thoughts were persistent and rampant. Thoughts of wanting to drive off a bridge or take over-the-counter medications began to haunt him. Finally, Katie recognized the symptoms of depression and brought John to see her doctor. The thought that John might become depressed was on his mother's radar and she finally disclosed that there was history of depression on his father's side: his paternal uncle was institutionalised.

Admission to a psychiatric facility was the ultimate stigma for John. He could not bring himself to be among "the crazy ones". He had very little contact with the baby and he didn't want her to come near the hospital. Caught

(continued)

between a depressed wife, a baby who needed him, and a set of parents who cared for him, John became increasingly despondent. Antidepressant medications were not very helpful for him. Suicidal ideations did not stop. He needed more aggressive treatment, and finally electroconvulsive therapy (ECT) was suggested. After about three unilateral ECTs, John's depression improved. Another three treatments were undertaken, and by the end of the sixth treatment, John was almost back to his baseline level of mood. His psychiatrist continued him on antidepressant medication and finally he was discharged home in the care of the specialist.

John and Katie accepted the help from both of their mothers and never looked back. By this point, they were no longer embarrassed to accept assistance from anyone. Katie's mother came to help her, as did her mother-in-law, with cooking, chores and the baby, while John and Katie rested as much as they could. The couple focused on the dynamics of their relationship, and worked very hard to come together to give Julie a stable life in the presence of parents who were psychologically stable and moving forward with their lives.

DSM-5 Diagnosis

Major Depressive Disorder with Peripartum Onset Specifier

This specifier can be applied for the most recent major depressive episode if the onset of mood symptoms occurs during pregnancy or in the 4 weeks following delivery. The diagnostic criteria for major depressive disorder are as follows:

Criteria A: Five or more of the following symptoms have been present during the same 2-week period and represents a change from previous functioning. At least one of the symptoms is either (1) depressed mood or (2) loss of interest or pleasure.

1. *Depressed mood most of the day, nearly every day, as indicated by either subjective report or observations made by others*
2. *Markedly diminished interest or pleasure in all or almost all activities most of the day nearly every day*
3. *Significant weight change when not dieting, or weight gain, or increase or decrease in appetite nearly every day*
4. *Insomnia or hypersomnia nearly every day*
5. *Psychomotor agitation or retardation nearly every day*
6. *Fatigue or loss of energy nearly every day*
7. *Feelings of worthlessness or excessive or inappropriate guilt nearly every day*
8. *Diminished ability to think or concentrate, or indecisiveness, nearly every day*
9. *Recurrent thoughts of death (not just fear of dying), recurrent suicidal ideation without a specific plan or a suicide attempt or a specific plan for committing suicide*

Criteria B: Symptoms cause clinically significant distress or impairment in social, occupational and other areas of functioning.

Criteria C: The episode is not attributable to effects of substance or another medical condition.

Criteria D: The occurrence is not better explained by schizoaffective disorder, schizophrenia, schizophreniform disorder, delusional disorder or other specified or unspecified schizophrenia spectrum and other psychotic disorders.

Criteria E: There has never been a manic or hypomanic episode.

Review of the Disorder

Introduction

Postpartum depression has been recognized in the mother for centuries. In clinical practice, occurrence of depression within 12 months after child birth is referred to as post partum depression. The mean prevalence of this complex psychiatric disorder is about 13 %. Depression in childbearing age is considered to be a public health burden. Currently, this psychiatric illness is well described in the DSM-5 under specified depressive disorder with peripartum onset. According to DSM-5, between 3% and 6% of women will experience onset of major depressive episodes either during pregnancy or in the weeks or months following delivery. Fifty percent of postpartum major depressive episodes actually begin prior to delivery, hence the collective use of the term *peripartum*. Many of these women also experience severe anxiety symptoms in addition to the depressed mood.

Biological markers of hormonal fluctuations unique to pregnancy and childbirth, thought to contribute to the etiology of depression in women are absent in the men. Nonetheless, the emotional upheaval leading to depressive psychopathology in fathers after the birth of a baby is a reality which is often overlooked. Thus, the depressive phenomenon in new fathers remains relatively unrecognized and undiagnosed. In the past decade, however, the occurrence of paternal postpartum depression is beginning to receive consideration among health-care providers. The stress of having a newborn generally affects both parents; dealing with the newborn requires adjustments on the part of the father as well. Due to a gradual shift in gender roles, fathers' involvement in child care has become more the norm in the western world. Many new fathers are hands-on dads; they often choose to take paternal leave in order to be available for their newborn babies. It appears that the birth of a child impacts the father just as much as it does the mother.

Epidemiology

Although current literature does not specifically define paternal postpartum depression, the diagnosis in clinical practice is based on the DSM-5 diagnosis of postpartum depression in the mother. Therefore, these are generally symptoms that can have their onset within the first 4 weeks' postpartum and can continue for 12 months' post-birth, as is commonly endorsed in women who suffer from postpartum depression. Based on current research, the incidence of paternal depressive symptoms is approximately 10% in postpartum fathers; this rate jumps to between 24% and 50% in fathers whose partners are experiencing postpartum depression. The wide statistical range may also have to do with inconsistency in research methodology, along with a lack of standardized guidelines and clinical heterogeneity.

Clinical Features

While there are many similarities between maternal and paternal depression after the birth of a newborn baby, literature shows, as does clinical experience, that the clinical manifestations of depression can be unique to fathers. Some specific symptoms such as episodes of anger, high levels of irritability, increased marital conflict as well as partner violence have been described by Kim and Swain (2007). Somatic presentations can be frequently vague, such as headache, nausea, diarrhoea, constipation or indigestion, which can be further confusing to primary clinicians as these symptoms overlap with multiple disorders. New fathers have been shown to display interpersonal behavioural changes that include social withdrawal, indecisiveness and irritability. These specific symptoms are often picked up by their partners, as the father's interactional pattern with the newborn child begins to change with developing depressive symptoms. These include withdrawal or avoidance (from social situations, work or family), indecisiveness, cynicism, anger attacks, affective rigidity, self-criticism, irritability, substance use, increased marital conflict, partner violence, somatic symptoms (e.g. indigestion, changes in appetite and weight, diarrhoea, constipation, headache, toothache, nausea and insomnia) and negative parenting behaviours (e.g. decreased positive emotions, warmth and sensitivity and increased hostility, intrusiveness and disengagement). Additional symptoms of paternal postpartum depression can include hypersomnia, psychomotor agitation or retardation, a lack of interest, concentration issues, other cognitive deficits such as memory issues and forgetfulness, anhedonia, the inability to enjoy the baby, worthlessness and guilt and, finally, in those few where the depression takes on a severe form, ongoing suicidal ideation. Characteristics of paternal depression are defined only in very few studies. For instance, only nine studies were found that used the term "paternal postpartum depression" to describe depression in new fathers when Goodman and colleagues reviewed the literature on paternal postpartum psychiatric disorders.

Risk Factors

It appears that maternal postpartum depression is the single most important risk factor that predicts paternal postpartum depression in the first year after childbirth. Male partners of women with depression feel less supported and experience increased stress during the postpartum period due to the demands of an infant, employment commitments and having to care for a depressed/anxious spouse. Additionally, this effect may be partly explained by the lack of emotional availability from the mother when the father starts to experience depressive symptoms. Lack of social support has been recognized as a risk factor for paternal PPD. With both parents in a state of emotional upheaval, neither one of them can draw comfort and/or a sense of support from the other. It is imperative to understand the implications of both parents suffering from postpartum depression as there is the risk for negative developmental outcomes in the baby. Fathers also play an important role when the mother is depressed by providing protection for the newborn baby. This ceases when fathers start to struggle with ongoing symptoms of low mood and are not able to establish the secure attachment that they could in the absence of a serious psychiatric illness. Depressed fathers tend to show less involvement in giving a bottle to the baby, playing with the baby, singing songs or bathing the baby. These are important developmental tasks not just for the infant, but also for the fathers, who tend to use these methods of being involved with the newborn as ways of attaching himself to the baby. Therefore, when these encounters do not occur, the father tends to feel guilty, less involved and more isolated. Several studies have found that there is a link between depressed fathers and poor developmental outcomes in newborn babies.

The Biopsychosocial Risk Factors for Paternal Postpartum Depression

DeMontigny conducted a study with a sample of fathers of infants whose average age was 11 months and who were exclusively breast-fed. They were compared with fathers with or without postpartum depression based on the EPDS. The results of this study showed that those fathers who were found to be depressed had experienced (i) perinatal loss in a previous pregnancy, (ii) parenting distress, (iii) a difficult infant temperament, (iv) dysfunctional interactions with the child, (v) decreased marital adjustment and (vi) perceived low parenting efficacy.

Among the biological risk factors that have been identified, very little research has shown exactly which biological predictors accompany paternal postpartum depression. However, levels of oestrogen, oxytocin and prolactin dysregulation have been identified as being correlated to maternal postpartum depression. Based on this existing knowledge, researchers have found that there might be an association between testosterone levels and paternal postpartum depression. Some researchers have suggested that paternal postpartum depression may be related to varying testosterone levels, specifically decreased testosterone over time, while their partner goes through pregnancy and postpartum changes. These researchers have suggested that this may result in better attachment towards the infant, lower aggression as well as better concentration with regard to parenting. Another study has shown that older men show a significant correlation between lower levels of testosterone and depression. Obviously, further studies are required in order to replicate these correlations. In the meantime, it appears that hormonal fluctuations have some association with paternal postpartum mood changes.

Another variable that has been implicated in paternal postpartum depression is an increase in the level of oestrogen. This could be seen as a hormone that enhances more active parenting after the birth of a child. Fleming and colleagues found that those fathers who were more engaged with their children had higher levels of oestrogen compared to those who were less engaged. It is possible then that that oestrogen dysregulation may play an important role in the development of postpartum depression in men.

Additionally, cortisol levels have been associated with paternal PPD. For instance, it is possible that lower levels of cortisol may regulate responses to stressful situations. Normally, high levels of this hormone are associated with high stress levels. For a mother, generally, higher levels of cortisol are associated with less depressed mood. Therefore, the lower levels of cortisol may account for father-infant bonding, with accompanying depressed mood. Finally, some of the older research on the role of vasopressin levels has found that they can contribute to paternal postpartum depression not unlike oxytocin levels in the mother, which increase after the birth of a child. Certain paternal behaviours such as protecting the infant could be due to the increase in levels of vasopressin. Therefore, it is possible that low levels of this hormone may contribute to difficulties in parenting behaviours and may be a risk factor for the onset of depression. Lastly, prolactin is one of the most important hormones responsible for instituting parental behaviours. Lower levels of prolactin could cause some fathers to adapt to ensuing parenthood, as suggested by Storey and colleagues.

Additional important risk factors for fathers include employment status, as well as paternal leave. In a Japanese study published in 2010, Nishimura and colleagues showed that fathers with temporary employment or unemployment were significantly more likely to be depressed. In addition, those who had a history of psychiatric treatment and those with unintended pregnancy were more prone to experiencing depressive illness in the postpartum period.

Societal support for new fathers underwent a concrete change in the last few years with the advent of paid paternity leave, which has been shown to be helpful for the development of a healthy family unit. Unfortunately, at the present time, the United States has no policy for paid paternity leave.

In many European countries, such as Finland, there has been a positive change associated with paternal leave for fathers. In Sweden, there has been encouragement for fathers to exercise their right to take leave after childbirth. There are several other countries where policies are in place for paternal leave. As a result, accumulating evidence shows that there are benefits to paternal leave including positive child outcomes. Given that there is a recent increase in fathers' involvement in parenting, it is important for society to focus on the added responsibility that fathers may face and encourage fathers to seek help when it is necessary.

Consequences for Infants and Children

The Avon Longitudinal Study of Parents and Children (ALSPAC) is a population-based study by Ramchandani, Stein, Evans and O'Connor that screened fathers for PPD at 8 and 21 months and assessed child behaviours at 3.5 years. The study showed the following three problem areas: emotional issues, conduct and hyperactivity. Findings of the study showed that paternal postpartum depression was associated with high scores in all three categories, more so for males than for females. Therefore, it appears that paternal postpartum depression can have both short- and long-term effects on the baby. Another study done by the same group in 2008 collected additional data up to 7 years in this population of children. They found that 12% of the children were diagnosed with attention deficit hyperactivity disorder, oppositional defiant/conduct disorder and/or anxiety and depressive disorders, if the father had postpartum depression. Therefore, based on these studies, it appears that paternal PPD may be more specifically related to behavioural and social problems in children. Another study by van den Berg and colleagues in 2009 showed a link between paternal postpartum depression and excessive infant crying in a cohort of fathers. Paulson and colleagues assessed both maternal and paternal depression, and development of language in the child at 24 months, as part of the early childhood longitudinal study birth cohort. The findings of this study showed that depression, in both mothers and fathers at 9 months, was associated negatively with parent-child activities, such as reading and singing songs.

What is clear from these studies is that the primary focus has been on maternal postpartum depression and its impact on the growing child. Now that we understand a little bit more about paternal postpartum psychiatric illness, specifically depression, it appears that the effect on the growing child in the milieu of both mother and father being depressed is significant and cannot be ignored. Some of the effects of untreated paternal and maternal depression include a higher risk of family stress, lack of bonding and incidents of both physical and emotional abuse, resulting in child psychopathology. Under such situations, clinicians must advocate for safety and protection of children. The primary care providers, as well as specialists who treat these parents, need to ensure that parents are referred to appropriate resources in the community, so as to prevent the potential negative and long-lasting consequences on the entire family.

Recommendations: How Do You Intervene?

Screening

There are a variety of different ways to screen for paternal postpartum depression, including the Edinburgh Postnatal Depression Scale (EPDS), the structured clinical interview (SCID) and/or the use of a standardized, structured interview as per DSM-5 in order to make a reliable diagnosis. The EPDS has been validated and used extensively for screening maternal postpartum depression. Several studies have reported the use of EPDS with fathers as well. The EPDS has also been translated into several different languages, such as Persian, Spanish, Portuguese and Greek, thus making it the most widely used screening instrument worldwide. The cutoff scores when screening for depression using the EPDS vary from culture to culture. These differences have not yet been documented well in fathers from various cultural groups. In western culture, for instance, men tend to be less expressive about emotional issues compared to women. Therefore, under these circumstances it would be incorrect to assume the same 12–13 cut-off point used for women with depressive illness. In clinical practice there is often a clear difference between males and females in the way that depressive symptoms are presented. Therefore, some researchers have suggested the cut-off point should be lowered by two to three points in order to correctly capture paternal postpartum depression.

Treatment

Prevention and Education

President Clinton reviewed mental health policies and directed the US Department of Health to institute support programmes to help men in their roles as fathers. The National Institute of Health and the National Institute of Mental Health led initiatives to assist in treatments of men as they handle the role of fatherhood. Men are less likely to report their mood and anxiety symptoms and do not seek help readily compared to women. Moreover, fathers suffering from postpartum depression do not receive prompt intervention because health-care professionals tend to minimize their symptoms. Some clinicians may feel uncomfortable about engaging in discussions about the father's mental health, especially when he becomes a new dad. Freitas and Fox allude to practice reflectivity whereby the therapists reflect on their own gender roles that can potentially block the assessment of postpartum psychiatric illnesses. For instance, a female therapist may want to somehow shield her male clients, and similarly, male therapists can be insensitive to the manifestation of symptoms as they see their male patients to be "strong". This then puts a greater burden on the suffering father as preconstructed barriers prevent him from being open and honest about his symptoms with his primary care providers; non-disclosure is further likely to increase his vulnerability. Fathers need to feel safe and comfortable in order to discuss their emotional instability without the fear of stigmatization. It is important for fathers not to feel judged. A family-centred approach in the context of the changing dynamic that takes into consideration the mother, father and the child can prove to be beneficial.

When the mother screens positive for depression, do not forget the father. Goodman and colleagues showed that around the 1 year postpartum mark, many fathers whose partners were depressed appeared to have symptoms of postpartum depression themselves. One explanation of this phenomenon is that the ongoing comorbidity with the suffering partner can eventually have a cumulative impact on the functioning of the father. Change in identity, the shifting of the relationship dynamic, as well as biological predisposition are some of the important factors that puts a father at higher risk for postpartum depression. Recognizing these risk factors will help facilitate prevention of depression and untoward consequences in the family as a whole. Routine education about the potential for depression in both parents after childbirth may facilitate earlier disclosure of symptoms. Irrespective of when the depression appears, what is really critical is to provide a multidisciplinary approach to fathers, mothers and the family as a whole.

Fathers whose partners are depressed have reported feelings of being isolated, overwhelmed, scared and stigmatized. Symptoms such as withdrawal, irritability, indecisiveness, anger, resentment, stress and fatigue have been associated with depression in fathers. There is a real urgency to understand the full extent of the changes that a father may experience after the birth. The primary care provider needs to be attuned to the father's experience of these various emotions which require careful clinical consideration. Professionals need to find a way for fathers to bond with the baby, explore the social construct of fatherhood, identify who their paternal role models are and define personal goals for fatherhood. Freitas and Fox advocate for systematic family assessment.

Their model of care offers approaches to treatment within a variety of different environments, with a maximal impact for fathers and families that are affected by postpartum paternal depression.

An Australian clinical psychologist, Dr. Habib, suggests providing psychoeducation to fathers around the changes that they might expect after childbirth. At our Reproductive Mental Health (RMH) Program, we follow a similar model by offering partner support groups run by our clinical/marital therapists on a weekly basis. We provide education around postpartum depression in fathers-only groups. The new dads are encouraged to talk about their depression in a more secure milieu and not feel embarrassed. Based on the feedback that we receive from fathers, these group educational endeavours have proven to be a positive method of intervention, not just for the fathers but for the family as a whole. Established in 1993 at the BC Women's Hospital, the RMH is a multidisciplinary clinic which consists of ten psychiatrists, two clinical counsellors, a nurse clinician, a marital therapist, a social worker, a project manager and two research assistants. We see up to 6,000 patients in the outpatient setting, offer consultation to the maternity inpatients and provide 24-h on call service.

It is not uncommon for fathers to attend prenatal appointments. Ideally, screening of paternal mood should take place during pregnancy. The third trimester of pregnancy for women is often fraught with heightened apprehension and increased emotional upheaval. Therefore, addressing the issues pertaining to overall vulnerability would not be out of place. Men are more than willing to open up, given the right circumstances and opportunities. Conjoint appointments with the expectant couple can encourage the father to talk about his concerns and fears; coming to terms with the new reality of parenthood is a challenge. While no measuring tools are available to screen men during their wives' pregnancies, we recommend ongoing dialogue between the primary health provider and both partners. The family physicians and/or obstetricians who see women through the pregnancy can engage in brief exchange of information with the attending fathers. Practicing a collaborative care model for fathers and mothers in the RMH Program has resulted in consistent and positive outcomes for the couple. Fathers who enrol in the group therapy sessions have expressed a high degree of satisfaction with type of intervention for coping with their own mood changes.

Lastly, the cross-cultural perspective of the father is important to take into consideration. Health-care personnel need to validate the legitimacy of paternal postpartum psychological struggles in the background of the cultural framework. Understanding the fears, the stigma or the shame attached to mental illness in a different cultural context is helpful in order to access appropriate recourse.

Management Strategies

Currently no clinical guidelines exist for the treatment of paternal PPD. Engaging new fathers in depression treatment and offering them the required support is still in its early stages. Emerging new knowledge appears to focus on the need for individualized treatment which targets management according to symptom presentation. Treatment of depression in new fathers should follow standardized treatment guidelines as they apply to depression in the general population. For treatment of moderate to severe depression, pharmacotherapy is recommended. Educating new fathers about tolerance to antidepressant medication remains a key factor in promoting adherence. Given that the side effect profile is high and onset of symptom relief takes place not earlier than 2 weeks, new fathers need to be aware of the short- and long-term gains related to this type of treatment. Sakado et al. suggest higher doses of antidepressant medications for those fathers who exhibit low paternal involvement because in their study, low efficacy with pharmacotherapy was found using traditional doses. If deemed to be suicidal, new fathers should be admitted to the hospital with appropriate interventions. Occasionally ECT may be required, as was the case with John, for complete symptom relief. If untreated, severe paternal PPD can have harmful consequences for family functioning.

Psychological treatments for mild to moderate depression include supportive psychotherapy, cognitive behaviour therapy (CBT), interpersonal therapy (IPT) and mindfulness-based interventions. These approaches to the management of paternal postpartum depression have been recommended by the NIMH Treatment of Depression Collaborative Research Program. Men generally respond well to tangible solutions, action-/goal-oriented problem solving and stress management techniques, including self-help programmes. As such, it is possible that cognitive behaviour therapies might be the most effective method of treatment for fathers to detect and understand their symptoms and be proactive in their own recovery. Online resources that explain different types of psychotherapies (e.g. by helping fathers understand terms such as CBT) are user-friendly ways for dads to learn more about these treatments. The effectiveness of group CBT in treating maternal postpartum depression is encouraging; a similar treatment model can be instituted in new fathers. Honey and colleagues incorporated psychoeducation, social skills training, pleasant skill activity scheduling, cognitive therapy and relaxation training exercises across twelve 2 h sessions. They included fathers in three of the sessions to provide information about maternal postpartum depression and suggestions for coping techniques and promoting social support. These group sessions were found to benefit the fathers; therefore, it is possible that they are more willing to engage in a group-based CBT approach. An earlier study by Gregg examined the effectiveness of group therapy for single fathers in Salt Lake City, Utah, where the focus was on dealing with social isolation and the negative aspects of a father's tendency to be a "super dad" as a compensatory mechanism to cope with the added responsibility of being a new father. Despite a fairly high study attrition rate, group therapy was found to be effective for new fathers.

IPT is the most rigorously studied therapy for maternal postpartum depression. This type of psychotherapy focuses on role transition, grief, interpersonal role disputes and interpersonal deficits. Similar areas of role conflict exist for fathers as for mothers; therefore, given the strong evidence base for this treatment in postpartum mothers, it is highly probable that IPT is effective in fathers suffering from postpartum depression as well. Mulcahy and colleagues did a randomized control trial looking at the effectiveness of group IPT versus treatment as usual for mothers with PPD. They found that group IPT significantly improved depression scores, as well as marital function and positive perception of the mother-infant relationship. Seeing as marital dysfunction is consistently a strong risk factor for both maternal and paternal postpartum depression, group IPT could be helpful for the father as well, especially given that expressing emotion is a significant fear for men during the perinatal period. Qualitative data on an Australian sample of postpartum depressed men identified escalating maladaptive patterns of behaviour, such as avoidance, emotional numbing, escape, etc. IPT as a treatment would help the father to refocus on his new role of providing for and protecting his family and adjusting to the increasing demands of fatherhood, such as helping his partner.

Mindfulness is often defined in the psychological literature as non-judgmental present-centred awareness. The practice of mindfulness assists by decreasing destructive thought patterns and creating introspection and allowing the mind to engage in self-reflection. Mindfulness-based stress reduction (MBSR) and mindfulness-based cognitive therapy (MBCT) are therapies that rely on mindfulness techniques such as body scan, meditation and breathing exercises. Mindfulness is meant to be practiced both formally and informally on a daily basis. Currently at the RMH, we are conducting a feasibility study assessing the efficacy of a mindfulness-based intervention in men at risk for experiencing postpartum depression and/or anxiety due to a clinical diagnosis in their partners. Studies show that mindfulness reduces stress, improves depression and anxiety symptoms and has an overall positive effect on relationships with significant others. Additionally, research suggests that paternal PPD could increase the likelihood of behavioural and emotional problems later in a child's life, that when fathers are not suffering from depression their involvement during the postpartum period can moderate the effects of maternal depression on child development and that the key predictor of paternal postpartum depression is a partner's postpartum mood disorder. As such, we predict that mindfulness training and therapy will be a helpful area of treatment for men who are at risk for, or who suffer from, postpartum depression. We are embarking upon investigating the effect of MBCT on fathers' overall well-being after childbirth, specifically examining the effects of such an intervention on marital harmony and parent-child interaction.

The biggest challenge that health-care providers are dealing with is the ability to engage the father in seeking treatment as they seem to do so far less than women. Therefore, methods that attract fathers to necessary resources are an important aspect of management. Creative strategies to increase fathers' awareness of this disorder include displaying information of paternal postpartum depression in waiting rooms of physician's offices and on bulletin boards in daycares, public libraries or health teaching clinics. Since prenatal classes are increasingly attended by expectant fathers, information about paternal postpartum depression displayed in these settings may be viewed by fathers as less threatening. Print resources that include specific contact information for counselling services are particularly valuable.

Although there is currently a dearth in research examining specific treatments for paternal postpartum depression, it is clear that there are many potential treatment routes that could benefit fathers who suffer from this disorder. Given the detrimental consequences – on both the individual and the family as a whole – of leaving men who suffer from PPD untreated, it is imperative that clinicians proactively screen for, as well as educate prospective dads on, the signs and symptoms of paternal PPD. In addition, treatments for paternal PPD should be made easily accessible for fathers in order to insure best possible outcomes. Providing readily accessible psychoeducational materials and treatments lessens the stigma and secrecy associated with paternal mental illness. This may help fathers to accept what they are feeling and take the necessary steps for recovery.

Take-Home Messages

1. The prevalence of paternal postpartum depression (PPPD) is estimated to be 10%, and the incidence of PPPD in men whose partners have postpartum depression (PPD) is reported to be 24–50%.
2. Under-diagnosis and under-treatment is the norm, due to stigma and shame, as well as societal expectations placed upon the new father.
3. While DSM-5 criteria for paternal postpartum depression do not currently exist, the present diagnosis is based on the maternal clinical manifestation of the same condition.
4. Screening of fathers whose partners are diagnosed with postpartum depression is recommended in order to identify paternal PPD.
5. Psychoeducation around paternal postpartum depression will reduce barriers and encourage participation in intervention.
6. Awareness of paternal PPD by primary health-care providers should be increased through the identification of biopsychosocial risk factors.
7. Treatment of paternal PPD involves pharmacotherapy, supportive psychotherapy, CBT and IPT.

References

1. American Psychiatric Association. Diagnostic and statistical manual of mental disorders (DSM-5®). American Psychiatric Pub, 2013.
2. Badker R, Misri S. Mindfulness-based therapy in the perinatal period: a review of the literature. BC Med J. 2017;59(1):18–21.
3. Berg S, Wynne-Edwards K. Changes in testosterone, cortisol, and estradiol levels in men becoming fathers. Mayo Clin Proc. 2001;76(6):582–92.
4. Cochran SV, Rabinowitz FE. Gender-sensitive recommendations for assessment and treatment of depression in men. Prof Psycol Res Pr. 2003;34(2):132.

5. Connell AM, Goodman SH. The association between psycho-pathology in fathers versus mothers and children's internalizing and externalizing behavior problems: a meta-analysis. Psychol B. 2002;128(5):746–73.
6. Davey SJ, Dziurawiec S, O'Brien-Malone A. Men's voices: post-natal depression from the perspective of male partners. Qual Health Res. 2006;16:206–20.
7. Demontigny F, Girard ME, Lacharité C, Dubeau D, Devault A. Psychosocial factors associated with paternal postnatal depression. J Affect Disord. 2013;150(1):44–9.
8. Fleming AS, Corter C, Stallings J, Steiner M. Testosterone and prolactin are associated with emotional responses to infant cries in new fathers. Horm Behav. 2002;42(4):399–413.
9. Freitas CJ, Fox CA. Fathers matter: family therapy's role in the treatment of paternal peripartum depression. Contemp Fam Ther. 2015;37:417–25.
10. Goodman JH. Paternal postpartum depression, its relationship to maternal postpartum depression, and implications for family health. J Adv Nurs. 2004;45:26–35.
11. Gregg C. Group work with single fathers. J Spec Group Work. 1994;19(2):95–101.
12. Grossman P, Nieman L, Schmidt S, Walach H. Mindfulness-based stress reduction and health benefits: a meta-analysis. J Psychosom Res. 2004;57:35–43.
13. Halle C, Dowd T, Fowler C, Rissel K, Hennessy K, MacNevin R, Nelson M. Supporting fathers in the transition to parenthood. Contemp Nurse. 2008;31(1):57–70.
14. Harvey I, McGrath G. Psychiatric morbidity in spouses of women admitted to a mother and baby unit. Br J Psychiatry. 1988;152:506–10.
15. Honey KL, Bennett P, Morgan M. A brief psycho-educational group intervention for postnatal depression. Br J Clin Psychol. 2002;41(4):405–9.
16. Karremans JC, Schellekens MPJ, Kappen G. Bridging the sciences of mindfulness and romantic relationships: a theoretical model and research agenda. Personal Soc Psychol Rev. 2015;21(1):29–49.
17. Kim P, Swain JE. Sad dads: paternal postpartum depression. Psychiatry. 2007;4(2):36–47.
18. Letourneau NL, Tryphonopoulos PD, Duffett-Leger L, et al. Support intervention needs and preferences of fathers affected by postpartum depression. J Perinat Neonatal Nurs. 2012;26:69–80.

19. Matthey S, Barnett B, Ungerer J, Waters B. Paternal and maternal depressed mood during the transition to parenthood. J Affect Disord. 2000;60(2):75–85.

20. Matthey S, Barnett B, Kavanagh DJ, Howie P. Validation of the Edinburgh postnatal depression scale for men, and comparison of item endorsement with their partners. J Affect Disord. 2001;64(2–3):175–84.

21. Melrose S. Paternal postpartum depression: how can nurses begin to help? Contemp Nurse. 2010;34(2):199–210.

22. Miniati M, et al. Interpersonal psychotherapy for postpartum depression: a systematic review. Arch Womens Ment Health. 2014;17(4):257–68.

23. Mulcahy R, et al. A randomized control trial for the effectiveness of group interpersonal psychotherapy for postnatal depression. Arch Womens Ment Health. 2010;13(2):125–39.

24. Musser AK, Ahmed AH, Foli KJ, Coddington JA. Paternal postpartum depression: what health care providers should know. J Pediatr Health Care. 2013;27:479–85.

25. Nishimura A, Ohashi K. Risk factors of paternal depression in the early postnatal period in Japan. Nurs Health Sci. 2010;12(2):170–6.

26. Paulson JF, Bazemore SD. Prenatal and postpartum depression in fathers and its association with maternal depression. JAMA. 2010;303:1961–8.

27. Paulson J, Dauber S, Leiferman J. Individual and combined effects of postpartum depression in mothers and fathers on parenting behavior. Pediatr Dent. 2006;118(2):659–68.

28. Ramchandani P, Stein A, Evans J, O'Connor TG. Paternal depression in the postnatal period and child development: a prospective population study. Lancet. 2005;365(9478):2201–5.

29. Ramchandani PG, O'Connor TG, Evans J, Heron J, Murray L, Stein A. The effects of pre- and postnatal depression in fathers: a natural experiment comparing the effects of exposure to depression on offspring. J Child Psychol Psychiatry. 2008;49(10):1069–78.

30. Rehel EM. When dad stays home too: paternity leave, gender, and parenting. Gend Soc. 2014;28(1):110–32.

31. Sakado K, Sato T, Uehara T, Sakado M, Someya T. Perceived parenting pattern and response to antidepressants in patients with major depression. J Affect Disord. 1999;52(1–3):59–66.

32. Schumacher M, Zubaran C, White G. Bringing birth-related paternal depression to the fore. Women Birth. 2008;21:65–70.

33. Seidman SN, Walsh BT. Testosterone and depression in aging men. Am J Geriatr Psychiatry. 1999;7(1):18–33.
34. Spector AZ. Fatherhood and depression: a review of risks, effects, and clinical application. Issues Ment Health Nurs. 2006;27(8):867–83.
35. Storey AE, Walsh CJ, Quinton RL, Wynne-Edwards KE. Hormonal correlates of paternal responsiveness in new and expectant fathers. Evol Hum Behav. 2000;21(2):79–95.
36. Tanaka S, Waldfogel J. Effects of parental leave and work hours on fathers' involvement with their babies. Evidence from the millennium cohort study. Community Work Fam. 2007;10(4):409–26.
37. Van den Berg M, van der Ende J, Crijnen A, Jaddoe V, Moll H, Mackenbach J, .. Verhulst FC: Paternal depressive symptoms during pregnancy are related to excessive infant crying. Pediatr Dent 124(1), 96–103, 2009.
38. Williams JMG, Kuyken W. Mindfulness-based cognitive therapy: a promising new approach to preventing depressive relapse. Br J Psychiatry. 2012;200:359–60.
39. Wilson S, Durbin E. Effects of paternal depression on fathers' parenting behaviors: a meta-analytic review. Clin Psychol Rev. 2010;30:167–80.
40. Wynne-Edwards KE. Hormonal changes in mammalian fathers. Horm Behav. 2001;40(2):139–45.

Chapter 3
Panic Disorder and Fatherhood: Anxiety in the Dad

Dad's Story: Clinical Vignette

Carlo and Raphaella had recently immigrated to Canada. Carlo's episodes of anxiety surfaced with his wife's unexpected pregnancy. He became increasingly panicky around Raphaella. Although stable on antidepressant medication, Raphaella relapsed with a diagnosis of postpartum depression after the baby's birth. Carlo's episodes of panic became more frequent and prolonged. After the birth of the baby, Carlo was found frantically opening windows at night because of breathlessness. He would become restless and tense, with complaints of being lightheaded and dizzy. He kept complaining of severe chest pain and was sweating profusely. The sense of dread and apprehension became so intense that he was convinced of dying of a heart attack. Raphaella had no choice but to call 911. An ambulance picked him up and took him to the nearest emergency room when the baby was 6 months old. The doctor's notes revealed that Angelo was suffering from acute panic attacks, triggered by the stress associated with the arrival of the new baby in his life. Additionally, relapse of depression was diagnosed

(continued)

© Springer International Publishing AG 2018
S.K. Misri, *Paternal Postnatal Psychiatric Illnesses*,
https://doi.org/10.1007/978-3-319-68249-5_3

which was thought to be precipitated by factors such as childbirth, immigration to a new country, exposure to a different culture and language barrier.

Angelo developed asthma around age 14. He had to be hospitalized several times because of acute asthmatic episodes. His mother, a well-meaning, anxious individual, tended to be over-protective of him because of his unpredictable health issues. During therapy sessions, it came to light that Angelo's move to Canada was not completely his choice. He felt pressured by Raphaella who had vacationed in Canada and fallen in love with the place. He was very anxious about starting a new life in a new country, as he was quite comfortable running his father's coffee business in Nicaragua. His father never really endorsed Angelo departing his homeland and felt upset by his son's decision to leave. Angelo recalled that his father was also an anxious man who used to have episodes of breathlessness, especially when he was in distressing situations. This was another reason why his mother continued to be over-protective of Angelo. Generally, she was focused on two family member: one being Angelo and the other being his father, Diego. Angelo and his father looked very similar, appeared to have similar personality characteristics, and dealt with stressful situation with physical symptoms of anxiety. His father worked hard over the years to be a financial success. He bought and sold coffee beans in great quantity and was hoping that Angelo would continue the family business and expand it. There was a lot of tension and anxiety around Angelo heading to Canada. His parents tended to make him feel guilty. Angelo had no way of coping with his own issues of conflict and his asthma attacks continued to increase. Many of these ongoing interpersonal conflicts between family members became obvious when he went into therapy and began to under-

(continued)

stand the connections, and the triggering and perpetuating factors. Angelo was able to be more focused and mindful to prevent further panic episodes. Whenever another full-blown anxiety attack seemed imminent, he would practice cognitive reframing in order to prevent and/or mitigate the panic attacks.

DSM-5 Diagnosis

Panic Disorder

Criteria A: Recurrent, unexpected panic attacks. A panic attack is an abrupt surge of intense fear or discomfort that reaches a peak within minutes, during which time four or more of the following symptoms occur:

- *Palpitations, pounding heart or accelerated heart rate*
- *Sweating*
- *Trembling or shaking*
- *Sensation of shortness of breath or smothering*
- *Feelings of choking*
- *Chest pain or discomfort*
- *Nausea or abdominal distress*
- *Feeling dizzy, unsteady, light-headed or faint*
- *Chills or heat sensations*
- *Paresthesia (numbness or tingling sensations)*
- *Derealization or depersonalization*
- *Fear of losing control or "going crazy"*
- *Fear of dying*

Criteria B: At least one of the attacks has been followed by 1 month (or more) of one or both of the following:

- *Persistent concern or worry about additional panic attacks or their consequences (e.g. losing control, having a heart attack, "going crazy")*

- *Significant maladaptive change in behaviour related to the attacks (e.g. behaviours designed to avoid having panic attacks, such as avoidance of exercise or unfamiliar situations)*

Criteria C: The panic attacks are not restricted to the direct physiological effects of a substance (e.g. a drug of abuse, a medication) or another medical condition (e.g. hyperthyroidism, cardiopulmonary disorders).

Criteria D: The disturbance is not better explained by another mental disorder (e.g. the panic attacks do not occur only in response to feared social situations, as in social anxiety disorder; in response to circumscribed phobic objects or situations, as in specific phobia; in response to obsessions, as in obsessive-compulsive disorder; in response to reminders of traumatic events, as in post-traumatic stress disorder; or in respect to separation from attachment figures, as in separation anxiety disorder).

Review of the Disorder

Introduction

Panic attacks bring on intense fear or discomfort which can reach its peak within minutes. Specifically, symptoms of losing control, going crazy or dying are very disconcerting and often cause people to seek help in the middle of the night. In Angelo's case, the episodes of panic related to the arrival of the baby were completely unexpected. Also, having not been diagnosed with these episodes when he lived in Nicaragua, their appearance in his early 30s came as a complete shock. He was aware that there was a lot of anxiety around coming to Canada; however, the early signs of headaches, sore neck and short fuse were not bothersome enough to take notice of. Angelo was aware that his asthma episodes might come back. Another scary issue with regard to the onset of his panic attacks was their occurrence in the middle of the night.

Angelo's first panic episode, where 911 was called, was in the middle of the night. Another symptom that was unexplainable was feelings of dizziness and numbness and tingling. A few times, he woke Raphaella with this very uncomfortable sensation; however, because the baby was so young and was waking up through the night, Angelo's own suffering and distress took a backseat. The particular night when the ambulance was called, he was experiencing a sense of unreality and felt that he was outside of his own body, looking at himself, with feelings of depersonalization.

While it is understandable that the birth of a baby can be an anxiety-provoking period for fathers, the onset of panic episodes is not frequently seen. In the context of extraordinary stressors, such as what Angelo was experiencing, the sensitivity to panic attacks appears to increase. Another factor that probably contributed to his panic attacks was smoking; many individuals appear to have an increase in panic episodes if they continue to smoke. This factor seems to be more common in females. When there is comorbidity with other mental disorders, including anxiety disorders, it appears that the panic episodes occur with a higher frequency. In the case of Angelo, although he did not have a prior history of mental health issues, it is quite possible that the stress related to his wife's depression may have been a triggering factor that set off the panic attacks. Sometimes other medical conditions, such as cardiovascular issues and asthma, can be correlated to panic attacks.

Epidemiology

As per the DSM-5, the 12-month prevalence of panic attacks in the general population is estimated in the United States and several European countries to be about 2% or 3% in adults and adolescents. Females are more frequently affected than males at a rate of 2 to 1. The gender differentiation occurs in adolescence, before the age of 14. It appears that prevalence rates decline as individuals age, possibly reflecting the diminishing severity to subclinical levels.

Barzega and colleagues investigated gender-related differences in the age of first panic attack/onset of disorder, familial history, comorbid conditions and occurrence of life events in the year preceding onset. One hundred and eighty-four participants were recruited at an outpatient department of which 39.1% were males. They had a primary diagnosis of panic disorder as per DSM-4. The researchers conducted semi-structured interviews to generate the DSM diagnosis and recorded the familial history of psychiatric disorders as well as history of stressful life events. The results showed a preponderance of females among patients with panic disorder. Additionally, those females with panic disorder also had higher educational levels compared to their male counterparts, and 19% of patients had first-degree relatives with a diagnosis of panic disorder. There was also a high percentage of panic disorder secondary to another Axis 1 disorder, and it is noteworthy that 9% of women had a history of bulimia. One of the most important findings of the study was that 74% of the participants had at least one stressful life event a year prior to the onset of their panic episodes. Moreover, the mean total score of all stressful life events and the mean single most stressful life event score were higher in female patients.

It appears that the process of immigration for Angelo was a very stressful life event which preceded the onset of panic episodes. The ultimate trigger appears to be the birth of the baby. He no longer felt he was in control of his life situation. The pregnancy was unexpected; there was a lot of tension between Raphaella and himself during the pregnancy. Angelo was afraid that he would not be a good father because he was fragile and vulnerable and felt that many of his dreams and aspirations were collapsing around him. In addition to his struggle of survival in a new country, the inability to speak the language was also a significant contributing factor. Raphaella spoke fluent English, whereas Angelo continued to be uncomfortable and had a lot of difficulty being in social situations. It is noteworthy that he did not use denial as a defence, but, instead, was open to intervention and was keen to get help. Often, this does not appear to be the case. Obviously, predisposition, personality traits and coping mechanisms are important factors in understanding who seeks help for panic disorder and who does not.

A study by Panayiotou and colleagues in 2014 examined the similarities and differences among individuals who met the strict screening criteria for panic disorder, GAD and social anxiety disorder. This study aimed to examine whether greater avoidance is associated with having symptoms of anxiety disorder, with greater psychological stress and/or anxiety comorbidity. The study included 457 adults, of which 162 were male, from a community sample in Cyprus. In this sample, 94 of the male participants had anxiety disorders, of which 38 met the criteria for panic disorder. The participants were assessed with the psychiatric diagnostic screening questionnaire (PDSQ) and the perceived stress scale, as well as the brief COPE and an AAQ questionnaire. The results showed that anxiety symptoms in all conditions had a significant positive correlation with coping, use of denial as a defence mechanism, self-distraction and behavioural disengagement. All conditions were significantly associated with experiential avoidance. The participants also appeared to score high on self-distraction compared to controls. The three most frequently used coping styles for those participants with panic disorder were planning, self-distraction and positive reframing. The conclusion of this study highlighted the role of avoidance as the paramount coping style and potential maintenance mechanism for anxiety pathology.

With the advent of parenthood, avoidance strategy is easy to fall back on, especially for new fathers. This is because in the first few weeks, if not months, there is a more intimate connection between the baby and its mother. Fathers are often onlookers and are not directly involved in the care of the baby. Therefore, avoiding being around stressors, specifically waking up at night to feed the baby, changing diapers, etc., can be easily avoided. This can increase the burden for the new mother and cause interpersonal conflicts. Therefore, understanding the coping style of somebody who is experiencing panic attacks, namely, fathers after the birth of a baby, is important to address, as over time it can lead to maladaptive coping mechanisms that can be repetitive, if not habitual. This can not only potentiate the psychopathology, but, as this paper showed, it can also help to maintain ongoing pathological interpersonal coping mechanisms within the family.

Clinical Features

Panic disorder is a psychiatric condition which can be easily misdiagnosed or have multiple symptoms that overlap with other medical and psychiatric disorders. For instance, a pounding heart or accelerated heart rate can occur in individuals with cardiovascular disease. Sweating is another symptom which is prevalent in many conditions, including cardiovascular disease and respiratory conditions, that can make accurate diagnosis confusing for health-care practitioners, especially if this is the only symptom that occurs consistently in individuals having panic attacks. Another interesting symptom often seen in patients with panic attacks is trembling or shaking. When panic attacks occur in older individuals, many neurological conditions are first considered before panic attacks are recognized. In a study by Corna in 2007 that examined the prevalence of risk markers for older adults in panic disorder, they found that 0.82% of older adults qualified for a diagnosis of panic disorder. In this particular population, the lifetime prevalence rate was found to be 2.45%. In the older population, interestingly enough, there were no gender differences found, unlike the younger population which had a female preponderance. Many of these older individuals had other comorbid symptoms of depression or social phobia. This study illustrates the frequency of panic attacks in an older population where misdiagnosis is easily possible. Another symptom, shortness of breath or smothering, can also be confused with respiratory conditions, especially those of asthma or chronic obstructive lung disease. Additionally, feelings of choking and chest discomfort and pain can also mimic respiratory pathology. With regard to gastrointestinal diseases, nausea and abdominal distress is one of the most common symptoms that can be misdiagnosed. In many individuals, severe panic attacks for a prolonged length of time can actually lead to diarrhoea. Finally, paresthesia or numbness and tingling can be very confusing, especially when there is a neurological workup being conducted in young adults with multiple symptoms. Finally, the fear of dying or "going crazy", which is sometimes the hallmark of panic attack, can be the central symptom that gets the attention of the attending clinician and points to the possibility of panic attacks. There are also culture-specific symptoms that include tinnitus and uncontrollable screaming or crying episodes. In postpartum practice, many women complain of "uncontrollable crying attacks" and/or anger attacks, which upon careful examination point towards classic panic episodes. In order to illustrate these specific symptoms of anxiety episodes, interviewing the patient carefully and in-depth will clear up any possible doubts about a diagnosis of panic attack. Often the clinical manifestations of agoraphobia occur in those with panic attacks. Agoraphobia is defined as a marked fear or anxiety about being in open spaces or enclosed spaces, using public transportation, or being outside of home alone. These individuals generally avoid situations that bring on fear or anxiety, because they are afraid in the event that they develop panic-like symptoms that it will be very embarrassing for them. The percentage of individuals with agoraphobia reporting panic attacks or panic disorder preceding the onset of agoraphobia ranges from about 30% to 50%. Therefore, it is not uncommon for some people to experience signs of anxiety and agoraphobia before the actual panic attacks occur. In addition, panic attacks are often associated with an increased likelihood of developing other anxiety disorders, depressive disorders and/or bipolar disorders.

In a 2014 study which identified parents with disabilities associated with different comorbidities, specifically depressive and phobic conditions, the researchers (Bonham and Uhlenhuth) examined 1,165 participants with panic disorder, with or without agoraphobia. They administered the Hamilton

Rating Scale for Depression and the Hamilton Rating Scale for Anxiety, along with the Sheehan Disability Scale. The researchers studied the extent of agoraphobia, worry, intensity of panic attacks and comorbidity. The results of this study showed that patients with panic attacks and comorbid agoraphobia, major depression and social phobia had increased disability in work, home and social functions. Those who had increased rates of agoraphobic avoidance, panic attacks and a number of situational panic attacks had higher scores of depression and anxiety on the Hamilton rating scales that eventually led to associated disability. The conclusion of the study was that the presence of agoraphobic avoidance and panic attack intensity and worry were associated with increased functional impairment and can serve as a warning for clinicians.

This is a particularly interesting area of concern, both for the new father and the new mother as they are going through a life-changing adjustment with the birth of a new baby. They are the primary care providers and have to not only protect their newborn but also in many ways advocate for their newborn. Avoidance, agoraphobia and comorbid conditions such as social anxiety can be a tremendous burden, both for the father and the mother. In families where both parents are suffering from psychiatric disorders, this burden increases. The functional impairment associated with ongoing panic disorder can be quite debilitating. Many new fathers, in clinical practice, have explained their discomfort around a newborn baby because the situation at home in some ways acts as a trigger for episodes of panic. It is not unusual for the fathers to spend long periods of time away from home, avoiding the situation that might cause anxiety. Therefore, early intervention is very important for these individuals who will continue on a chronic course if it remains untreated.

Recurrent, unexpected panic attacks constitute Panic Disorder. Usually, they occur in the context of another anxiety disorder or other mental conditions and/or medical conditions. In the case of Angelo, he suffered from asthma and so the panic attack specifier fit his case. However, eventually, because of the recurrence of panic attacks over the next 6 months, he more accurately fit the criteria for panic disorder. Panic disorder refers to recurrent, unexpected panic attacks, and the term "recurrent" means that there is more than one unexpected panic attack. Unexpected panic attacks refer to those episodes for which there is no obvious cue or trigger at the time of the occurrence and that such an episode can occur from out of the blue, such as when a person is relaxing or emerging from sleep. With Angelo, it appears that at first his panic attacks were unexpected, and eventually, because they were triggered by stressful situations at home with the baby and his wife, they became more recurrent and thus met the criteria for panic disorder. Another important consideration that needs to be understood is the anticipatory anxiety or worry about another panic attack and the maladaptive changes which represent attempts to minimize these consequences. Luckily, this was not the case with Angelo. Prior to his developing worry about the next panic attack, he received treatment, and the panic attacks eventually disappeared. However, when panic attacks have continued for this long, the possibility of them returning in the future with any stressors is usually high. It is important to understand the risk factors associated with panic disorder.

Risk Factors

A variety of risk factors for panic disorder exist, including environmental, genetic, physiological and temperamental vulnerability. The literature reports that traumatic experiences early in childhood, especially physical and sexual abuse, are significant psychosocial risk factors for the onset of many anxiety disorders. Interpersonal stressors related to physical well-being, negative experiences with illicit or prescription drugs and disease or death in the family are some other additional environmental factors that will make an individual vulnerable to panic attacks. In a study by Bandelow and colleagues, early traumatic events, parental attitude, family history and birth risk factors were investigated with regard to their association with panic disorder. They recruited outpatients with panic disorder and matched controls. Both groups were interviewed with a standardized questionnaire. The results of this study showed that events leading to separation from a parent, such as death, major hospitalization of the father, illness of the child, unemployment of the father or employment of the mother, were associated with panic disorder. Other important factors included the death of the mother or being an only child. Having a large, extended family in the same house during childhood appeared to be a protective factor against panic disorder. Whereas alcoholism, violence and sexual abuse in parents were more frequently reported in those with panic disorder, these patients also reported that their parents were less loving and paid little attention to them compared to those in the control group. This study concluded that certain traumatic environmental factors were significantly correlated to the development of panic disorder in later life. It appears that unfavourable parental attitudes and familial history were found to correlate with the development of panic disorder, and a familial transmission of anxiety disorders was suggested. However, this data is retrospective and the results should be interpreted with caution. Nonetheless, in clinical practice, it is not uncommon to see many of these environmental factors as predisposing factors for manifestation of panic disorder later on in adult life. Specifically sexual or physical abuse, parental attitudes and genetic predisposition are some of the risk factors that appear to be frequently present in this population. In Angelo's case, it appears that being an only child was one of the risk factors, while having his aunts and uncles around in the same household was probably a protective factor. His father's inability to be supportive when he left the country appears to be the single most important trigger for the onset of panic disorder.

With regard to the genetic and physiological predisposition, multiple genes appear to confer vulnerability to the onset of panic disorder. However, the exact genes and their implication at this point remain unknown. There also appears to be an increased risk for panic disorder among the offspring of parents with anxiety, depressive and bipolar disorder. Respiratory disturbances such as asthma are also associated with panic disorder, in terms of past history, comorbidity and family history.

There is an abundance of literature examining the genetic vulnerability to panic disorder. A very interesting study in 2017 by Deckert and colleagues examined the GLRB allelic variations associated with anxiety conditions. In particular, they investigated the neurogenic pathways to panic disorder. They performed a genome-wide association study examining the molecular genetics of panic disorder with and without agoraphobia. There were a number of volunteers in whom the complicated genetic study went beyond the classical diagnostic genotypes and investigated which neuromechanisms were linked to behaviours. The researchers summarized that the evidence for GLRB-allele variation may contribute not only to rare neurological disorders but also to the risk of milder anxiety disorders such as panic disorder and agoraphobia by increasing the startle response. Studies are being conducted on the epigenetics of anxiety disorders which show that while knowledge regarding the contributions of epigenetic processes in the development of behavioural disorders, including anxiety disorders, is evolving, it is still in its infancy. Most researchers so far implicate genes regulating the HPA axis, neurotransmitter systems and neuroplasticity in the etiology of anxiety disorders. In addition to genetic vulnerability factors, personality and behavioural characteristics seem to moderate between life events and the development of panic disorder. This was demonstrated in a study by Klauke in 2010, where life events in those with panic disorder were studied. A literature review was conducted by researchers where they examined the life events that contributed to the pathogenesis of panic disorder. The results showed that threat, interpersonal loss and health-related life events were found to be main stressors for panic disorder. Abuse, loss and separation events were additional contributing factors. Comorbidity with major depression was an important additive factor. Genetic makeup, however, appears to set the biological vulnerability. These are the individuals at higher risk and in whom stressful life events are encountered. Therefore, high anxiety sensitivity and neuroticism may be mediating factors that appear to increase vulnerability to panic disorder.

Panic Disorder Comorbidity

In clinical practice, panic disorder mimics many other medical conditions. The most common medical issue that a patient may present at the hospital with is feeling like they are having an acute heart attack with a sense of doom and gloom. Another common condition is hyperthyroidism or other endocrine disorders. Thirdly, a concurrence with asthma is not uncommon, and finally panic attacks can mimic a medical condition such as multiple sclerosis. Often emergency room visits are overutilized by patients with panic disorder. With regard to the gender distribution of comorbidity, it appears specifically in males in the form of substance use and personality disorders that accompany panic attacks, whereas with females, it appears that anxiety, depression and eating disorders tend to coexist with panic attacks. With regard to additional psychiatric disorders, bipolar disorder, other anxiety disorders and especially agoraphobia often accompany panic disorder. These individuals tend to have onset in childhood, with separation anxiety being one of the common symptoms that is displayed, especially when a child leaves home to go to school. Many patients, especially during adolescence, are found to be at a higher risk for suicide when they are experiencing frequent, moderately strong panic attacks. Early childhood trauma is seen as being an important risk factor, along with increased vulnerability or sensitivity.

With regard to childbirth, this is considered an important and stressful life event, which can lead to the onset of panic attacks. This was the case with Angelo who had onset of panic attacks after the birth of his child. In addition, he did have comorbid asthma. In those individuals who are asthmatic, any hyperventilation can cause further broncho-constriction, thereby leading to worsening of the asthma. Eventually, in the case of Angelo, worsening of his asthmatic symptoms and exacerbation of panic attacks took on a cyclical occurrence which had to be stopped with cognitive behaviour therapy. In particular, breathing training becomes an important part of therapy when treating patients with asthma and panic attacks.

In conclusion, understanding the high degree of comorbidity with medical conditions, treatment of panic disorder in the context of pre-existing medical illness is important. Sometimes, engaging in cognitive behaviour therapy without the knowledge of a medical condition can lead to worsening of the existing illness. Conversely, many clinicians are not able to make the connection between the birth of a baby and occurrence of panic attacks, as when males do appeal for help, this diagnosis is easy to miss in the context of other medical conditions.

Impact of Paternal Panic Attacks on Children

Research shows that anxiety disorders run in families with an underlying predisposition. Whether or not parents who have panic disorder pose a risk for the subsequent appearance of this illness in their children remains uncertain. What is clear is that there appears to be a general anxiety proneness in children whose parents are affected by anxiety disorders. In one study conducted by Biederman and colleagues, the purpose was to evaluate whether an underlying familial predisposition is shared by all anxiety disorders and/or whether panic disorder and major depression have a familial link. The researchers compared four groups of children. The first group of 179 children were the offspring of parents with panic disorder and comorbid depression. The second group consisted of 29 children who were the offspring of parents with panic disorder without comorbid major depression. The third group were the offspring of parents with major depression without comorbid panic disorder and numbered 59. The final group of 113 children were the offspring of parents with neither panic disorder nor major depression. The results of this study showed that parental panic disorder, regardless of comorbidity with major depression, was associated with an increased risk for panic disorder and agoraphobia in the offspring. Parental major depression, regardless of comorbidity with panic disorder, was associated with an increased risk of social phobia, major depression, disruptive behaviours, behaviour disorders and poorer social functioning in offspring. These children were also at risk for separation anxiety and multiple (i.e. two or more) anxiety disorders. This study concluded that the findings confirmed previous results which documented a significant association between the presence of panic disorder and major depression in parents and psychopathology and dysfunction in their offspring.

Another related study, conducted by Rosenbaum and colleagues, aimed to examine the specificity of an association between behavioural inhibition and anxiety. They recruited parents with comorbid panic disorder and depression or stand-alone PD or depression and assessed their children for behavioural inhibition. Behaviour inhibition is a temporal construct which refers to the consistent tendency of some children to demonstrate fear and withdrawal in novel situations. In this particular study, the researchers based the definition of behavioural inhibition on certain behaviours in the children, which included smiles, spontaneous comments or exhibition of fears. The authors found the children whose parents had both panic disorder and depression were at a particularly high risk for behaviour inhibition. This was evident across all measures of behavioural inhibition. In addition, children of parents with only one of the disorders had intermediate levels of behavioural inhibition that were indistinguishable from the controls. In other words, the conclusion of the study was that when panic disorder and major depression occur in a comorbid manner, there is more conference of familial risk between parental panic disorder and child behavioural inhibition. In clinical practice, the importance of recognizing the comorbidity between the two illnesses in parents is essential in order to provide a safe environment for the child to grow up in. It is also important to ensure that there are enough protective factors present for the father to be able to cope with the appearance of the illness at some later time in the presence of certain stressful situations. In the case of Angelo, for instance, it appears that when he was growing up, his father may have suffered from anxiety episodes and/or possibly depression that was not treated. Growing up in an environment filled with tension and anxiety can eventually lead not only to the onset of panic attacks in childhood or adolescence but also to the perpetuation of the disorder if the environmental stressors remain unchanged.

In an interesting study by Vogels and colleagues performed in 2008, the rearing behaviours of fathers of anxious children were examined. The investigators found that fathers of anxiety-disordered children were less supportive of their partners, dominated conversations relative to their partners and were less autonomy encouraging. They also seemed to have a negative impact on the mother's rearing behaviours. In other words, children who are anxious also impact the parental dynamic. For instance, in this study, the fathers and mothers of anxiety-disordered children were more controlling than parents of the control group. Interestingly enough, the mother's anxiety status was not associated with different rearing behaviours in both parents. This study concluded that father's anxiety status seemed to make a difference in raising an anxious child.

These studies showed two things, one is that there is clearly a genetic predisposition towards panic attacks and it follows a familial vulnerability. The other is that environmental stressors can also explain the genesis and maintenance of panic disorder. Stressful life events also contribute to the onset or timing of the illness, along with many other medical comorbidities and psychiatric disorders. The important part of prevention cannot be understated, as early intervention of the disorder can preclude the development of the illness in a chronic manner later on in life.

Treatment Recommendations: How Do You Intervene?

Pharmacological Treatment of Panic Disorder

Tricyclic antidepressants were one of the first studied medications which reported efficacy in treating panic disorders. Pharmacotherapy not only prevents occurrence of panic attacks but also reduces and eliminates the anticipatory anxiety as well as phobic avoidance. In adequate doses, an antidepressant effect can be seen with most antidepressant medications. Presently, all selective serotonin reuptake inhibitors (SSRIs) have been found to be effective in the treatment of panic disorder. There have been several positive placebo-controlled randomized trials supporting the efficacy of a variety of different SSRIs which include sertraline, paroxetine, escitalopram, citalopram, fluoxetine and fluvoxamine. There is some evidence pointing to escitalopram being superior to citalopram in the treatment of panic disorder. Medications that should be carefully avoided during an acute treatment of panic attacks include bupropion; many patients on bupropion (or Wellbutrin) will have worsening of panic attacks.

Serotonin and norepinephrine reuptake inhibitors (SNRIs) have also been found to be effective in the treatment of panic disorder, with most studies having been conducted on extended release venlafaxine. In some refractory patients, MAOIs have been shown to be effective, especially in individuals with phobic anxiety. MAOIs are not in recent use, however, because of their potentially lethal interaction with certain foods. Benzodiazepines can be useful in the short term, if there is education for the acute onset of panic attacks which are severe and continuous. Sometimes introducing an SSRI in these patients can activate their anxiety. Clinically, many physicians will start these patients on a short-term benzodiazepine trial and then add the SSRIs and titrate them upwardly. The issue with benzodiazepines is their high potential for addiction and abuse, but if monitored closely, these medications do have a place in the treatment of panic attacks. Co-prescription of benzodiazepines and SSRIs is common. Due to the worry of abuse, many physicians are hesitant to use this particular class of medications. This can be harmful for those who may benefit from short-term intervention and long-term gain until the SSRIs begin to take effect. Studies have shown that discontinuation of medications inadvertently can produce relapse in a large number of patients. Therefore, follow-up on a regular basis, no matter which antidepressants they are on, is essential. Another important component of patient adherence is to educate them about panic disorder and to accept responsibility for their treatment. Therefore, educating people about why they need to take medications to control their psychological symptoms is an essential exercise.

Studies in patients who have responded to acute treatments reveal that there is an advantage to staying on active medication compared to switching, or to placebo, for at least 6 months. In addition, findings of acute treatment indicate that a proportion of responders steadily increases over time.

The addition of group CBT may be beneficial to non-responders. A study done by Craske aimed to evaluate the relative effectiveness of medication with CBT versus medication alone for panic disorder in primary care settings. The participants in these studies include primary care patients with panic attacks, who were males between the ages of 17 and 70. They were randomized either to CBT or expert medication recommendation or treatment as usual. Assessments were given at baseline, 3 months and 12 months post-treatment. The results of this study showed that those patients who received both CBT and anti-panic medications fared better at 3 months compared to those who were just treated with medications alone. These findings were also sustained, and even enhanced, at 12 months post-study. There was a general preference for CBT. Those who selected medications were less severe at baseline and were more likely to have been taking medications at baseline. The conclusion of this study was that CBT and medications were shown to be superior compared to medications alone in the treatment of panic disorder. Primary care physicians are encouraged to consider CBT in addition to medications.

Psychological Treatment of Panic Disorder

Although there is robust evidence with regard to the effectiveness of CBT alone, or in combination with medications, this type of treatment in Canada, the United States and the UK is underused for a variety of reasons. These include restricted access to mental health professionals who provide this kind of treatment, unfamiliarity with the nature and efficacy of CBT for clinicians who recommend it and the affordability of such treatments. Therefore, many clinicians have limitations with regard to referring patients for cognitive behaviour therapy. This type of treatment emphasizes psychoeducation about panic. It also aims to correct misconceptions with regard to panic symptoms and cognitive restructuring, which focuses on correcting distortions and understanding the exposure to bodily sensations that bring about fear.

In addition, in vivo exposure and interoceptive exposure to fear situations are therapeutic techniques used to treat panic attacks. Interoceptive exposure techniques were studied by Botella where they examined the efficacy of virtual reality exposure (or VRE) in the treatment of panic attacks. They chose patients who fit DSM-5 criteria for diagnosis of panic disorder, with or without agoraphobia in males. These patients were interviewed and given fear and avoidance scales, Panic Disorder Severity scales as well as anxiety sensitivity indices, agoraphobia subscales and depression inventories. Many other scales were given, including maladjustment and clinical global impression. Pre- and post-treatment follow-ups were done. Participants were randomized to in vivo exposure (IVE) or virtual reality exposure (VRE) or control. Virtual reality (or VR) is an emerging technology that allows simulation of different real situations in a tridimensional computer-generated environment. The user can interact with this environment as though it was real. The idea of using such technology is that by interacting in this kind of setting, the patient learns to accept this environment as the real world. This is also an alternative way of treating those individuals who cannot tolerate in vivo treatment. Furthermore, in contrast to in vivo exposure, VR allows for accurate graduation of exposure to the fear, object or situation.

The results of Botella's study showed that VRE was just as effective as in vivo treatment and was maintained for about 12 months following the end of treatment. Patient satisfaction was very high, as they felt that VRE treatment was useful. The conclusion of this study was that there were many promising results with regard to the efficacy of VR treatment. While it is not meant to be used as replacement for in vivo, it is certainly a new way to apply a well-established older technique.

The specific contribution of techniques of exposure, cognitive therapy, relaxation training and breathing retraining has not yet been clearly established. A meta-analysis by Sanchez-Meca analyzed the efficacy of psychological intervention, which included a combination of exposure, relaxation training and breathing techniques. The treatments were then classified in a variety of different combination categories to tease apart the best effect. The conclusion of the study was that the optimal treatment found in the literature was in vivo exposure with relaxation training or breathing retraining. Additionally, the inclusion of homework and follow-up programmes was very beneficial. In the case of Angelo, ten sessions focusing on exposure in vivo with relaxation training were very helpful. Additional treatments included interpersonal psychotherapy as well as support within the marriage as he began to improve with proper therapeutic interventions. In addition to cognitive behaviour therapy, Angelo also stayed on a small dose of escitalopram, 10 mg daily, which he continued to take for the next year or so. Combining different modalities of treatment finally led to almost complete remission of symptoms. Research has shown that when psychotherapy and antidepressants are combined, they are definitely superior to either one of the monotherapies. Also, generally, it has been found that combination therapy has a much lower drop-out rate compared to combination therapy. Studies have also shown that if antidepressant medication continues, then the relapse prevention is high in these individuals, which is what Angelo experienced. At the 6-month mark, when he discontinued escitalopram, his symptoms came back, and an educational session with his family doctor and with his psychologist led to an improvement in his compliance and adherence with treatment. His family doctor was reticent to start Angelo on benzodiazepines because of long-term concerns of being on this particular medication. What it comes down to is that even if Angelo was to take lorazepam and/or clonazepam for a short length of time, eventually relapse prevention would occur with the help of cognitive behaviour therapy, which is best in combination with antidepressants.

Take-Home Messages

1. The 12-month prevalence of panic disorder in the general population is estimated to be around 2–3%.
2. Stressful life events, such as new parenthood, have been found to precipitate the onset of this disorder.
3. Panic disorder is a psychiatric condition which can be easily misdiagnosed or has multiple symptoms that overlap with other medical and psychiatric disorders.
4. Often the clinical manifestations of agoraphobia occur in those with panic attacks.
5. Sexual or physical abuse, parental attitudes and genetic predisposition are risk factors that appear to be frequently present in those with panic disorder.
6. Parental panic disorder is associated with an increased risk for panic disorder and agoraphobia in the offspring.

7. Treatment of panic disorder involves a combination of pharmacotherapy and psychotherapy, such as SSRIs in combination with CBT with exposure. Early intervention is key.

References

1. American Psychiatric Association. Diagnostic and statistical manual of mental disorders (DSM-5®). Washigton, DC: American Psychiatric Pub; 2013.
2. Aschenbrand SG, Kendall PC, Webb A, et al. Is childhood separation anxiety disorder a predictor of adult panic disorder and agoraphobia? A seven-year longitudinal study. J Am Acad Child Adolesc Psychiatry. 2003;42(12):1478–85.
3. Bandelow B, Späth C, Tichauer GÁ, et al. Early traumatic life events, parental attitudes, family history, and birth risk factors in patients with panic disorder. Compr Psychiatry. 2002;43(4):269–78.
4. Barzega G, Maina G, Venturello S, et al. Gender-related differences in the onset of panic disorder. Acta Psychiat Scand. 2001;103(3):189–95.
5. Batinić B, Trajković G, Duisin D, et al. Life events and social support in a 1-year preceding panic disorder. Psychiatr Danub. 2009;21(1):33–40.
6. Biederman J, Faraone SV, Hirshfeld-Becker DR, et al. Patterns of psychopathology and dysfunction in high-risk children of parents with panic disorder and major depression. Am J Psychiatry. 2001;158(1):49–57.
7. Bögels SM, Bamelis L, van der Bruggen C. Parental rearing as a function of parent's own, partner's, and child's anxiety status: fathers make the difference. Cogn Emot. 2008;22(3):522–38.
8. Bonham CA, Uhlenhuth E. Disability and comorbidity: diagnoses and symptoms associated with disability in a clinical population with panic disorder. Psychiatry J. 2014;2:1–8.
9. Botella C, García-Palacios A, Villa H, et al. Virtual reality exposure in the treatment of panic disorder and agoraphobia: a controlled study. Clin Psychol Psychother. 2007;14(3):164–75.
10. Carlbring P, Nilsson-Ihrfelt E, Waara J. Treatment of panic disorder: live therapy vs. self-help via the internet. Behav Res Ther. 2005;43(10):1321–33.

11. Cassiello-Robbins C, Conklin LR, Anakwenze U, et al. The effects of aggression on symptom severity and treatment response in a trial of cognitive behavioural therapy for panic disorder. Compr Psychiatry. 2015;60:1–8.
12. Corna LM, Cairney J, Herrmann N, et al. Panic disorder in later life: results from a national survey of Canadians. Int Psychogeriatr. 2007;19(6):1084–96.
13. Craske MG, Golinelli D, Stein MB, et al. Does the addition of cognitive behavioral therapy improve panic disorder treatment outcome relative to medication alone in the primary-care setting? Psychol Med. 2005;35(11):1645–54.
14. Deckert J, Weber H, Villman C, et al. GLRB allelic variation associated with agoraphobic cognitions, increased startle response and fear network activation: a potential neurogenetic pathway to panic disorder. Mol Psychiatry. 2017;22:1–9.
15. Ewing DL, Dash S, Thompson EJ, et al. No significant evidence of cognitive biases for emotional stimuli in children at-risk of developing anxiety disorders. J Abnorm Child Psychol. 2016;44(7):1243–52.
16. Furukawa TA, Watanabe N, Churchill R. Combined psychotherapy plus antidepressants for panic disorder with or without agoraphobia. Cochrane Libr. 2009;188:1.
17. Greenslade JH, Hawkins T, Parsonage W et al. Panic disorder in patients presenting to the emergency department with chest pain: prevalence and presenting symptoms. Heart Lung Circ. 2017;26:2–7.
18. Hendrick V. Postpartum panic disorder in a new father. Am J Psychiatry. 2002;159(1):150.
19. Klauke B, Deckert J, Reif A, et al. Life events in panic disorder—an update on "candidate stressors". Depress Anxiety. 2010;27(8):716–30.
20. Nelson BD, Perlman G, Hajcak G, et al. Familial risk for distress and fear disorders and emotional reactivity in adolescence: an event-related potential investigation. Psychol Med. 2015;45(12):2545–56.
21. Nieto SJ, Patriquin MA, Nielsen DA, et al. Don't worry; be informed about the epigenetics of anxiety. Pharmacol Biochem Behav. 2016;146:60–72.
22. Ozkan M, Altindag A. Comorbid personality disorders in subjects with panic disorder: do personality disorders increase clinical severity? Compr Psychiatry. 2005;46(1):20–6.

23. Panayiotou G, Karelka M, Mete I. Dispositional coping in individuals with anxiety disorders symptomatology: avoidance predicts distress. J Contextual Behav Sci. 2014;3(4):314–21.
24. Rosenbaum JF, Biederman J, Hirshfeld-Becker DR, et al. A controlled study of behavioral inhibition in children of parents with panic disorder and depression. Am J Psychiatry. 2000;157(12):2002–10.
25. Roy-Byrne PP, Uhde TW, Post RM. Effects of one night's sleep deprivation on mood and behavior in panic disorder: patients with panic disorder compared with depressed patients and normal controls. Arch Gen Psychiatry. 1986;43(9):895–9.
26. Sánchez-Meca J, Rosa-Alcázar AI, Marín-Martínez F, et al. Psychological treatment of panic disorder with or without agoraphobia: a meta-analysis. Clin Psychol Rev. 2010;30(1):37–50.
27. Steinman SA, Hunter MD, Teachman BA. Do patterns of change during treatment for panic disorder predict future panic symptoms? J Behav Ther Exp Psychiatry. 2013;44(2):150–7.
28. Watanabe N, Churchill R, Furukawa TA. Combination of psychotherapy and benzodiazepines versus either therapy alone for panic disorder: a systematic review. BMC Psychiatry. 2007;7(1):18.

Chapter 4
Generalized Anxiety Disorder in Fathers After a Newborn: When Worry Takes Over

---

Dad's Story: Clinical Vignette

Jay had separation anxiety as a child. During his adolescence, he watched his parents fight. He used to dread the evenings when his father would come home drunk and be verbally or physically violent towards his mother. Helpless and afraid, he would hide in his bedroom with rapid heartbeat and chest pains. He grew up a worrier. He worried about his own safety as well as that of his mother. She eventually left the marriage and raised Jay as a single parent. Jay's contact with his father remained sporadic throughout his life. Starting very early in his life, he dreamed of having 'the perfect family'.

During his teens, Jay kept busy by playing on the school football team and kept himself occupied with part time jobs and schoolwork. Throughout his adulthood, although restless and on edge compared to his peers, Jay appeared to cope with his anxiety fairly adequately and functioned well. He held a steady job in his local

(continued)

© Springer International Publishing AG 2018
S.K. Misri, *Paternal Postnatal Psychiatric Illnesses*,
https://doi.org/10.1007/978-3-319-68249-5_4

Municipal office as a bookkeeper and had been living together with Mary for 2 years. She was a teller in their local bank and was content with her life in general. They loved the outdoors; camping and kayaking and hiking were some of the activities they enjoyed. Their life together was stable and predictable.

All of this changed drastically when Mary lost their newborn baby. Their little girl died 2 months after birth due to a rare medical condition. Devastated, Jay coped with this loss by becoming intensely involved in Mary's grief. He always wanted to have a family and could not wait to be a father. He started to worry about the possibility of never becoming a father. The couple planned the second pregnancy soon after. Jay became very apprehensive and nervous throughout Mary's subsequent pregnancy. He was constantly concerned with its outcome and was up at night with various irrational thoughts. Over the ensuing weeks, Jay started to experience physical symptoms of anxiety such as occasional diarrhea, stomach discomfort, and breathlessness.

Unfortunately, the second pregnancy ended in tragedy as well; Mary had a stillbirth. Jay became distraught with escalating anxiety; the anticipation of another loss haunted him relentlessly. Finding it difficult to control this worry, he was keyed up and on edge all the time. Mary would watch him pacing restlessly through the night. Tense and irritable, Jay could not stop ruminating over yet another loss. Impossible to access and communicate with because of his uncontrollable worries, Jay became a challenge to live with. This ongoing noncommunicative behavior affected Mary's mood; she become sad and distant. She also realized that Jay's anxiety was beyond the scope of being normal. Mary contacted their doctor for immediate assistance. Although reluctant to seek help at first, Jay was relieved to visit the doctor, who diagnosed him with Generalized Anxiety Disorder (GAD).

(continued)

Jay was referred by his family doctor to see a psychologist for Cognitive Behaviour Therapy (CBT). In therapy sessions, Jay was able to explore his early childhood experiences, his coping skills, and other contributing factors which led to the precipitation of uncontrollable worries, eventually meeting the criteria of GAD. He also joined yoga classes, went for long walks and practiced mindfulness. He is now working to strengthen his coping skills that will help him manage his stress.

DSM-5 Diagnosis

Generalized Anxiety Disorder (GAD)

Criteria A: Excessive anxiety and worry (apprehensive expectation), occurring more days than not for at least 6 months, about a number of events or activities (such as work or school performance).

Criteria B: The individual finds it difficult to control the worry.

Criteria C: The anxiety and worry is associated with at least three of the following physical or cognitive symptoms:

- *Restlessness, feeling keyed up or on edge*
- *Being easily fatigued*
- *Difficulty concentrating or mind going blank*
- *Irritability*
- *Muscle tension*
- *Sleep disturbance (difficulty falling or staying asleep or restless, unsatisfying sleep)*

Criteria D: The anxiety, worry or physical symptoms cause clinically significant distress or impairment in social, occupational or other important areas of functioning.

Criteria E: The disturbance is not attributable to the physiological effects of a substance (e.g. a drug of abuse, a medication) or another medical condition (e.g. hyperthyroidism).

Criteria F: The disturbance is not better explained by another medical disorder (e.g. anxiety or worry about having panic attacks in panic disorder, negative evaluation in social anxiety disorder [social phobia], contamination or other obsessions in obsessive-compulsive disorder, separation from attachment figures in separation anxiety disorder, reminders of traumatic events in post-traumatic stress disorder, gaining weight in anorexia nervosa, physical complaints in somatic symptom disorder, perceived appearance flaws in body dysmorphic disorder, having a serious illness in illness anxiety disorder or the content of delusional beliefs in schizophrenia or delusional disorder).

Review of the Disorder

Introduction

Excessive, disproportionate worry which interferes with psychosocial functioning characterizes Generalised Anxiety Disorder (GAD). The content of these worries can change from time to time, ranging from the simplest issues pertaining to daily chores, to health, work, finances or disasters. The worries seem to be more than what is warranted for the actual events, often resulting in severe apprehension; the individuals expect the worst when there is often no reason for concern. A person who is preoccupied with these irrational worries cannot "switch them off" and tends to ruminate over them in an unhealthy manner. Individuals with GAD find it difficult to focus or concentrate as the worries are generally distracting and persistent, leading to fatigue and exhaustion; they may complain of their mind "going blank". Sufferers are often imprisoned in their own thoughts and are unable to engage in social or occupational functioning. Symptoms of irritability, insomnia and being on edge can cause further impairment.

In many individuals, GAD needs no precipitant. For Jay, his earlier struggle with separation anxiety was a risk factor in the eventual manifestation of GAD, although his GAD symptoms were manageable during his early adulthood. Their onset was triggered by grief and loss related to two consecutive failed pregnancies. His symptoms were intense and pronounced due to the distressing and painful life circumstances which simply overpowered him, rendering him dysfunctional. Jay began to be overconcerned about Mary, as he was about his mother who was a constant source of anxiety for him. Jay relived the familiar, marked discomfort associated with watching his mother with his abusive father. When Mary was traumatized, both mentally and physically; she had a C-section. Pervasive anxiety set in and the worry cycle began with catastrophic thinking and reassurance-seeking behaviours.

Epidemiology

Worldwide, about 3.6% of the general population is affected by GAD. Although commonly encountered, postpartum anxiety in new fathers is not written about with the same frequency as postpartum depression. Currently, there are very few studies which examine paternal postpartum anxiety, in specific GAD. Leach and colleagues reviewed 43 papers on expectant/new fathers to examine the prevalence rate of anxiety in cross-cultural sample and found the rates to be variable, anywhere between 2.4% and 18%. This variability could be due to a number of factors such as the country where the study was conducted, the type of symptom scale used or the cut-off points for diagnosis. For instance, in the Australian sample, the prevalence rate of GAD was about 12.2%, whereas in the UK sample, there was a reported rate of 3.4%. It appears that the course of anxiety symptoms remained fairly constant throughout their partner's pregnancy with a potential decrease in the postpartum period for most of the studies reviewed by Leach et al. This review denotes that anxiety disorders are common for men, both in the prenatal and the postnatal period. Clearly, GAD is not specific to new mothers only.

An interesting study on paternal anxiety by researchers in Hong Kong examined 622 expectant fathers in early pregnancy, late pregnancy and 6 weeks postpartum. A variety of different psychological instruments were included in this study: the Anxiety Subscale of the Hospital and Depression Scale (HADS), the Multidimensional Scale of Perceived Social Support scale, the Rosenberg Self-Esteem Scale, the Work-Family Conflict Scale, the Kansas Marital Satisfaction Scale as well as the EPDS. The results of this study showed that a significant portion of expectant fathers experienced anxiety during the entire perinatal period. The study also showed that the probability of paternal anxiety increased as the pregnancy proceeded, peaking at about 6 weeks postpartum (a prevalence of 11.6–14.25%). Finally, marital stress, lower self-esteem, low social support, high levels of work/family conflict and having a partner with depression or anxiety were identified as psychosocial risk factors that could trigger these anxiety symptoms.

Sympathetic response to pregnancy (couvade syndrome) is more likely to be seen when an expectant father is not involved in prenatal classes or is not allowed to be present in the delivery room. In recent years, active paternal involvement is expected, especially in western society. Transitioning to fatherhood, fear of the unknown and providing hands-on care to their newborn often lead to anxiety in the new dad. The extent of anxiety in an expectant father was studied by Matthey and colleagues, an Australian research group who recruited 408 women and 356 men antenatally and followed the couples in the postpartum period. A variety of measures were used to determine the presence of major and minor depression, panic disorder, acute adjustment disorder with anxiety and finally specific phobias. Acute adjustment disorder with anxiety was the most prevalent disorder found in fathers, with a rate of approximately 30%. In the presence of acute adjustment disorder with anxiety or panic disorder, the rates of comorbid depression increased by approximately 30–100% in this sample. What was also of interest is that the wives of these men were two to three times more likely to meet the criteria for depression and anxiety. Therefore, the results of this study show that it is important to assess for depression as well as anxiety in both parents.

Clinical Features

To meet the DSM V criteria for GAD, the excessive, irrational worry must occur for more days than not for a minimum duration of 6 months. In clinical practice, typically, the acute and unsettling anxiety presentation in new mothers meets all of the GAD qualifiers required by the DSM other than the criteria of duration. Adhering strictly to this definition can potentially lead to under-diagnosis and exclude a considerable number of women from accessing timely help. Researchers now accept 1–2 months' duration to be sufficient in order to consider a diagnosis of maternal postpartum GAD provided they meet the other criteria. In Matthey's study, the dads diagnosed with adjustment disorder and anxiety actually met the GAD criteria, but their illness was of less than 6 months' duration.

Similarly, in another study, Wynter and her research group used modified criteria to define GAD, i.e. that the sufferers did not have symptoms for 6 months. They investigated a community sample in Victoria, Australia, for the period prevalence of postpartum depression, anxiety and adjustment disorders in women as well as their male partners. They excluded populations that were at higher risk, for instance, single parents and/or non-English-speaking populations. Measures used included EPDS and the Composite International Diagnostic Interview (CIDI) at 6 months postpartum. Their results showed that 4.1% of men had at least one anxiety disorder, whereas 17.4% met the criteria for acute adjustment disorder with anxiety or modified GAD. They also found that anxiety was more common than depression in this sample. The results of this study show that the GAD symptoms are common among new fathers in the first 6 months postpartum. The rates of paternal anxiety appear equal to those found in maternal anxiety in some studies.

It appears that paternal anxiety is more prevalent during pregnancy compared to the postpartum period. Many fathers experience decreases in their anxiety once the baby is born. In one study, second-time fathers were shown to experience the same level of anxiety as first-time fathers. Therefore, the continuation of intervention through every pregnancy might be warranted. In addition, a one-time assessment might actually limit the detection of paternal anxiety at other points of time during pregnancy. Assessing fathers' mental health problems starting from early pregnancy is recommended. Preliminary evidence shows that including fathers early in the assessment period can reduce the risk of postnatal anxiety. In their recent study, Rowe and colleagues showed that men continue to report feeling excluded and irrelevant in both prenatal and postnatal health care. Therefore, it is essential to include both partners in discussions during obstetrical care. Formal supports need to be available to men when required. Given its high prevalence rate, there is greater need for clinical attention as well as research focus on paternal anxiety. The potentially detrimental effects of anxiety on the partner and the child are another reason as to why early intervention should be easily obtainable by these fathers. The successful transition of a man into a paternal role should not be taken for granted or undermined.

Risk Factors

Often, the screening tools that are available to detect depression also detect anxiety. A lower cut-off score will likely give more indication of anxiety mixed with depressive symptoms, both in mothers as well as fathers. Some studies are looking at the risk factors for psychological symptoms which may be gender specific and how a father's manifestations of distress might be captured earlier on in the pregnancy as well as postpartum. However, in general, studies in postpartum paternal anxiety still appear to be rare. Luoma and colleagues attempted to examine the paternal, maternal, infant and family factors associated with the occurrence of anxiety and depressive symptoms in fathers of infants. The researchers asked both parents to complete the EPDS at a routine check-up at 4, 8 or 18 months postpartum. They used lower cut-off scores for fathers, around 5–6, and for mothers, 7–8. In total, 194 families were involved in this study. The results were interesting as 21% of the fathers and 24% of the mothers scored above the cut-off points for depression and anxiety. Moreover, both the paternal and maternal factors of employment, perceived mental health, work-related problems and quality of their relationship predicted high levels of paternal anxiety, and there was a strong association between partners' symptoms. Additionally, having two or more children was also linked to higher paternal EPDS scores. Previous studies have shown that being a single father and having older children is often associated with postnatal general psychological distress in fathers. Interestingly enough, in this study by Luoma, infant factors were not statistically significant when it came to the association with paternal anxiety or mood symptoms. The important message from this study is that the whole family system should be considered when there are concerns about either of the parents' psychological well-being. The postpartum stage is a time of transition for both parents, and the rapidly changing role of fatherhood increases the direct impact on the father when a child is born. Postpartum depressive and anxiety symptoms in fathers are strongly associated with similar symptoms in mothers. While the psychological distress of the father may be less risky to an infant at this point in time than the mother's, given that the infant spends more time on average with the mother, this study shows that the father's psychological problems may have more impact as children mature and the father's role becomes increasingly important.

Another interesting aspect of risk factors for anxiety in pregnancy and postpartum includes how a father's adverse background could be linked to the appearance of clinical symptoms. In a study recently published in 2015, by researchers in Oslo, Norway, it was shown that there is a significant correlation between retrospectively reported adversity in early childhood and feelings of depression and anxiety during all time points in pregnancy. Memories of their own early childhood may influence how these fathers see themselves as caregivers. A lot of these men were found to have early interpersonal relationship difficulties, which triggered anxiety later on in their adult lives. Some of them also had issues relating to their own fathers as appropriate role models, and hence their own understanding of what fatherhood ideally would be like was not consolidated at some level. Therefore, in the process of transitioning to fatherhood, many of these individuals may continue to experience conflicts between their own experiences as a child and how that might impact their ability to be an effective father. In general, fathers with poor self-esteem, little family support and a high level of marital dissatisfaction appear to be at a higher risk for experiencing anxiety. Predictors of anxiety focusing on transitional experiences for prospective fathers include feelings of unreality, insufficiency and inadequacy. These could negatively impact their role as a father. It is important in understanding that childhood experiences which are negative among fathers-to-be make them increasingly vulnerable to experiencing depression and anxiety during their partner's pregnancy. The experience of being a father could bring back memories of their own adverse childhoods for those who have not had a closure of their early incurred trauma; this may influence how they see themselves as caregivers for their own children. Also, contemporary fathers may likely use their own fathers as role models for the current pregnancy, which may then lead to feelings of anxiety and depression if their own early life experiences were adverse. Therefore, research on fathers' depressive and anxious feelings during pregnancy and the related risk factors is important to pursue.

Alcohol abuse has been linked to depression and anxiety in men. Although depression and anxiety is more prevalent among women compared to men, it appears that one of the ways that men handle themselves when experiencing emotional distress is to drink excessively. Therefore, it is important to study the effects of alcohol use during pregnancy as far as the partners are concerned. For most fathers, especially first-time fathers, the fear of the unknown in dealing with the various aspects of pregnancy can be a challenge. Currently, the prevalence and correlates of perinatal anxiety and alcohol dependence in men have not been researched enough. A recent study by Fisher and colleagues examined the relationship between pregnancy and alcohol misuse by men in the northern part of Viet Nam. The researchers enrolled 231 men whose wives were at just over 28 weeks of gestation or were mothers of newborns. They were interviewed using DSM-4 criteria, and self-reporting questionnaires were also given to them. The fathers were found to have depressive disorders and GAD, which occurred comorbidly. There was no difference with regard to prevalence rates during pregnancy and/or in the immediate postnatal period. While problematic alcohol use was prevalent, it was most common among men who had completed just 9 years of formal education. These men were also more likely to be unskilled workers living in the poorest households. Therefore, the conclusion of this study was that common mental disorders and alcohol dependence were prevalent but were unrecognized in men from northern Viet Nam whose wives were pregnant or had just given birth. It is noteworthy that this prevalence appears to be different from higher-income and well-resourced Asian countries.

Not much is known about the effects of paternal anxiety on a growing child. The role of controlling parents and how they may negatively impact childhood anxiety disorders has been written about by researchers in the past. Overcontrolling parents are those who show a high level of intrusion and vigilance – they show less warmth and acceptance and appear to be more critical and rejecting of their children. It is unclear whether it is the child who elicits or triggers these kinds of behaviours in parents or whether parental anxiety is responsible for a child's anxiety symptoms. It is possible that parents who are anxious themselves may be more rejecting towards their children. In other words, the direction of this relationship remains unclear. There are a variety of different explanations behind this specific behaviour. For instance, they may be overprotective because they are reducing their own anxiety by exposing their child to less danger. They may also be controlling their own fright reaction by directing and criticizing. In a study done by Bögels, the researchers examined the parenting behaviours of 121 children who were referred to a clinic with a diagnosis of an anxiety disorder. These children ranged in age between 8 and 18 years. The aim of the study was to examine the parenting behaviours based on the parents' own partners as well as their child's anxiety status. The findings were interesting. This is because fathers with anxiety appeared to exert more control and rejection towards their growing children. Children with anxiety also had fathers who were less supportive of their partners. The study also found that fathers with anxiety were more dominant in conversation. Finally, in families where the fathers were anxious, both parents' rearing appeared to be negatively impacting the child's development. The findings of this study showed that the father's anxiety status seemed to have a more pervasive effect on child-rearing compared to the mother's status. In the past, studies have looked extensively at the impact of maternal anxiety on the child. Therefore, this particular study increases the awareness of how a father's mental health may impact the rearing of his child. The study also shows that those fathers who are anxious themselves will be less effective in their role of autonomy and encouragement, which in turn could result in anxiety in the child. Also, paternal anxiety appears to indirectly affect the child through the mother's rearing practices. For prevention and treatment, intervention for childhood anxiety disorder must involve the role of the father's anxiety as it appears to play a significant part in the behaviour of the child. Fathers may have a different contribution to make when it comes to coping with their child's anxiety. Likely, fathers who suffer from anxiety may not be able to parent their child in the way that a child would normally expect, for instance, engaging in more physical interaction or more active play, etc. It may be interesting and important to investigate the causal relationship between paternal anxiety and child-rearing.

Recommendations: How Do You Intervene?

Treatment Interventions

The focus of any treatment intervention when it comes to the parents should include providing education and support to fathers, especially if the partner is breast-feeding. This is because often fathers feel left out and do not have an avenue to freely express their anxiety. Evidence shows that the capacity to parent effectively depends on the mental health status of not just the mother, but also the father. The shifting role of new fathers now goes beyond just the joy and excitement that fatherhood brings about, as there is an increase in the responsibility that is bestowed upon the new father. Therefore, their contribution with regard to the ongoing emotional, mental and physical development of the child has to be acknowledged and recognized. The importance of actively trying to reduce paternal anxiety during the child's formative years has to be addressed. Different factors can impact the appearance of anxiety in fathers; change in interpersonal relationships, increased financial responsibility, limited emotional availability of the partner and redefining self-identity can be some of the issues that come up normally for each and every father as he journeys through this transition. This is especially true for first-time fathers who have no idea what to expect when they become a parent. Very few hospital-based antenatal programs recognize the contribution of the father, especially emotionally, in the first few weeks, if not months, of infancy. It is generally the mother who bonds intimately with her breast-fed infant, thus making the father feel inadequate and non-participatory.

In a study by Tohotoa, the researchers in Australia focused on examining the impact of a father-inclusive intervention for perinatal anxiety and depression. This repeated measure cohort study conducted as a part of a larger randomized controlled trial (RCT) took place across eight maternity hospitals and enrolled 533 expectant fathers. The primary focus of the intervention was to provide education and support to fathers of breast-feeding partners with the aim of increasing both initiation as well as duration of breast-feeding. The fathers were part of a group educational program which was led by a male facilitator during pregnancy and 6 weeks postpartum. The results showed that the intervention group had less self-reported anxiety from baseline to 6 weeks postpartum compared to those fathers who were in the control group. They felt more confident in their ability as a parent, had resources for problem solving and had good social support systems.

It appears that some fathers do experience anxiety prior to the birth of their child, but around 6 weeks postpartum, this anxiety reduces rapidly, especially if they are provided with information and strategies for increasing their knowledge, thereby potentially reducing the risk of onset of postnatal anxiety. With timely intervention, these fathers feel more confident about their paternal role and are more helpful in preventing sleep deprivation in their partners, which in turn will help these breast-feeding mothers. Finally, it is important for the fathers to "fit" their baby into their lifestyle and have the opportunity to discuss their experiences with other fathers. So, a venue where such interaction is possible should be made available to them, whether at the maternity clinic or community centres. Just like mothers, it appears that fathers also value access to other fathers and want to talk about the learning curve in coping with their own anxiety as it arises. Fathers need to be made aware of early infant contact as well as sharing with other males about their own fathering practices. The importance of communication between fathers can be an important support for the mothers. In addition, if there is a previous history of depression or anxiety in the fathers, they can be flagged in the postnatal period for close follow-up by public health and/or primary care physicians. Resources that would be available for these men obviously vary from country to country, as would the availability of appropriate personnel and funding. What is clear is that educating fathers with relevant information can act as an important intervention that could potentially reduce the risk of anxiety in the father, the mother and the child and ensure the well-being of the family as a whole.

An innovative method of intervention for reducing anxiety and promoting satisfaction with regard to parenting for fathers was studied in first-time Filipino fathers by using music therapy. In this prospective study, 98 first-time fathers were included, of whom 50 were allocated to the music group and 48 were in the control or nonmusic group. This study was designed to assist in determining the effect of music on anxiety in first-time Filipino fathers after childbirth. A variety of different soothing and calming music was used, mostly classical. Earlier studies have shown that music that is slow and flowing, with low notes consisting mostly of stringed instruments and a maximum volume level of 60 decibels is preferred. This music was recorded in five multimedia players with accompanying headphones. Subjects chose the music they liked from a list of pre-recorded music selections. Paternal anxiety was measured using a scale called the State-Trait Anxiety Inventory or STAI, before and after exposure to music. The satisfaction with the childbirth experience was also measured on a visual analog scale. The results of this study showed that 30 min of music intervention significantly lowered anxiety scores and increased satisfaction scores during their partners' labour and delivery. The anxiety scores in the nonmusic group increased. The music group also reported high satisfaction with labour and birth and was able to support their partner during labour. This interesting study provides empirical evidence to support the use of music as a strategy in reducing anxiety and promoting satisfaction in first-time fathers. Also, a reduction in anxiety scores could have been attributed to the anxiolytic effects of music in general. Besides, such an intervention is inexpensive, it is not invasive and it is easily administered. Finally, it will be interesting to see if such an intervention would be applicable in other situations in the postpartum period to see if a reduction of anxiety is possible for fathers as well as mothers. Another study where a group-based parent training program was undertaken to improve parental psychosocial health showed that such training led to significant short-term improvements in paternal stress compared to the control group.

Although the appearance of anxiety disorders is common in the adult years, many of these individuals feel anxious all of their lives with waxing and waning of symptoms in a chronic manner. The development and course of this condition underscores the need to provide services for men once they are identified as sufferers, offer prevention and set guidelines for intervention. GAD symptoms can be debilitating and can affect a father's ability to effectively assume his paternal role. Studies thus far show that paternal anxiety has a potential negative impact on the father/child relationship. One study showed that early in the postpartum period, especially around 6 weeks after the birth of the baby, the dads seemed to experience a peak in their anxiety symptoms. Excessive anxiety has been found to prevent the father from being an emotional support and/or be physically present for his partner who is transitioning to the maternal role. As such, it is essential that supports are put in place to help new fathers address their anxiety.

Take-Home Messages

1. Prevalence rates of anxiety with expectant and postpartum fathers are significant. They are as high as maternal anxiety. When they occur comorbidly with depression, these rates increase significantly.
2. It is important to assess both anxiety and depression in expectant parents and offer anxiety management strategies that might prove beneficial for the whole family.
3. Paternal risk factors for anxiety include employment status, work-related problems, quality of the partner relationship and perceived mental health issues.
4. The whole family system should be considered when there are concerns about either parent's psychological well-being.
5. Alcohol dependence often goes unrecognized in men whose wives are pregnant or have just given birth.
6. Paternal anxiety negatively affects child development.
7. Early treatment intervention aimed at psychoeducation and social support is highly encouraged.

References

1. Alibekova R, Huang JP, Lee TS, et al. Effects of smoking on perinatal depression and anxiety in mothers and fathers: a prospective cohort study. J Affect Disord. 2016;193:18–26.
2. Armstrong KA, Khawaja NG. Gender differences in anxiety: an investigation of the symptoms, cognitions, and sensitivity towards anxiety in a nonclinical population. Behav Cogn Psych. 2002;30(2):227–31.
3. Ayers S, Wright DB, Wells N. Symptoms of post-traumatic stress disorder in couples after birth: association with the couple's relationship and parent–baby bond. J Reprod Infant Psychol. 2007;25(1):40–50.
4. Barlow J, Smailagic N, Huband N, et al. Group-based parent training programmes for improving parental psychosocial health. Cochrane Libr. 2014;2014(5):1465–858.
5. Bögels SM, Bamelis L, van der Bruggen C. Parental rearing as a function of parent's own, partner's, and child's anxiety status: fathers make the difference. Cogn Emot. 2008;22(3):522–38.
6. Boyce P, Condon J, Barton J, et al. First-time fathers' study: psychological distress in expectant fathers during pregnancy. Aust N Z J. 2007;41(9):718–25.
7. Bradley R, Slade P, Leviston A. Low rates of PTSD in men attending childbirth: a preliminary study. Br J Clin Psychol. 2008;47(3):295–302.
8. Diemer GA. Expectant fathers: influence of perinatal education on stress, coping, and spousal relations. Res Nurs Health. 1997;20(4):281–93.
9. Dugas MJ, Freeston MH, Ladouceur R, et al. Worry themes in primary GAD, secondary GAD, and other anxiety disorders. J Anxiety Disord. 1998;12(3):253–61.
10. Figueiredo B, Conde A. Anxiety and depression in women and men from early pregnancy to 3-months postpartum. Arch Womens Ment Health. 2011;14(3):247–55.
11. Fisher J, Tran TD, Nguyen TT, et al. Common perinatal mental disorders and alcohol dependence in men in northern Viet Nam. J Affect Disord. 2012;140(1):97–101.
12. Helle N, Barkmann C, Ehrhardt S, et al. Postpartum anxiety and adjustment disorders in parents of infants with very low birth weight: cross-sectional results from a controlled multicentre cohort study. J Affect Disord. 2016;194:128–34.

13. Koh YW, Lee AM, Chan CY, et al. Survey on examining prevalence of paternal anxiety and its risk factors in perinatal period in Hong Kong: a longitudinal study. BMC Public Health. 2015;15(1):1131.
14. Labrague LJ, McEnroe-Petitte DM. Use of music intervention for reducing anxiety and promoting satisfaction in first-time Filipino fathers. Am J Mens Health. 2016;10(2):120–7.
15. Leach LS, Christensen H, Mackinnon AJ, et al. Gender differences in depression and anxiety across the adult lifespan: the role of psychosocial mediators. Soc Psychiatry Psychiatr Epidemiol. 2008;3(12):983–98.
16. Leach LS, Poyser C, Cooklin AR, et al. Prevalence and course of anxiety disorders (and symptom levels) in men across the perinatal period: a systematic review. J Affect Disord. 2016;190:675–86.
17. Liber JM, van Widenfelt BM, Goedhart AW, et al. Parenting and parental anxiety and depression as predictors of treatment outcome for childhood anxiety disorders: has the role of fathers been underestimated? J Clin Child Adolesc Psychol. 2008;37(4):747–58.
18. Luoma I, Puura K, Mäntymaa M, et al. Fathers' postnatal depressive and anxiety symptoms: an exploration of links with paternal, maternal, infant and family factors. Nord J Psychiatry. 2013;67(6):407–13.
19. Matthey S, Barnett B, Howie P, et al. Diagnosing postpartum depression in mothers and fathers: whatever happened to anxiety? J Affect Disord. 2003;74(2):139–47.
20. Meadows SO, McLanahan SS, Brooks-Gunn J. Parental depression and anxiety and early childhood behavior problems across family types. J Marriage Fam. 2007;69(5):1162–77.
21. Mitte K. Meta-analysis of cognitive-behavioral treatments for generalized anxiety disorder: a comparison with pharmacotherapy. Psychol Bull. 2005;131(5):785.
22. Möller EL, Majdandžić M, Bögels SM. Parental anxiety, parenting behavior, and infant anxiety: differential associations for fathers and mothers. J Child Fam Stud. 2015;24(9):2626–37.
23. Parfitt Y, Ayers S. Postnatal mental health and parenting: the importance of parental anger. Infant Ment Health J. 2012;33(4):400–10.
24. Pilkington P, Milne L, Cairns K, et al. Enhancing reciprocal partner support to prevent perinatal depression and anxiety: a Delphi consensus study. BMC Psychiatry. 2016;16(1):23.

25. Skari H, Skreden M, Malt UF, et al. Comparative levels of psychological distress, stress symptoms, depression and anxiety after childbirth—a prospective population-based study of mothers and fathers. BJOG. 2002;109(10):1154–63.
26. Skjothaug T, Smith L, Wentzel-Larsen T, et al. Prospective fathers' adverse childhood experiences, pregnancy-related anxiety, and depression during pregnancy. Infant Ment Health J. 2015;36(1):104–13.
27. Somers JM, Goldner EM, Waraich P, et al. Prevalence and incidence studies of anxiety disorders: a systematic review of the literature. Can J Psychiatr. 2006;51(2):100–13.
28. Teetsel RN, Ginsburg GS, Drake KL. Anxiety-promoting parenting behaviors: a comparison of anxious mothers and fathers. Child Psychiatry Hum Dev. 2014;45(2):133–42.
29. Tohotoa J, Maycock B, Hauck YL, et al. Can father inclusive practice reduce paternal postnatal anxiety? A repeated measures cohort study using the hospital anxiety and depression scale. BMC Pregnancy Childbirth. 2012;12(1):75.
30. Turton P, Badenhorst W, Hughes P, et al. Psychological impact of stillbirth on fathers in the subsequent pregnancy and puerperium. Br J Psychiatry. 2006;188(2):165–72.
31. Wee KY, Skouteris H, Richardson B, et al. The inter-relationship between depressive, anxiety and stress symptoms in fathers during the antenatal period. J Reprod Infant Psychol. 2015;33(4):359–73.
32. Wittchen HU. Generalized anxiety disorder: prevalence, burden, and cost to society. Depress Anxiety. 2002;16(4):162–71.
33. Wynter K, Rowe H, Fisher J. Common mental disorders in women and men in the first six months after the birth of their first infant: a community study in Victoria, Australia. J Affect Disord. 2013;151(3):980–5.
34. Zelkowitz P, Milet TH. The course of postpartum psychiatric disorders in women and their partners. J Nerv Ment Dis. 2001;189(9):575–82.
35. Zerach G, Magal O. Anxiety sensitivity among first-time fathers moderates the relationship between exposure to stress during birth and posttraumatic stress symptoms. J Nerv Ment Dis. 2016;204(5):381–7.

Chapter 5
Obsessive-Compulsive Disorders in New Fathers: Feeling Out of Control

Dad's Story: Clinical Vignette

Dad's Story

Matt was known throughout high school as a scholar. At university, he began to check and recheck his work several times a day, a habit he deemed to be more an asset than a hindrance. He decided to pursue a career in computer technology, confident that he would excel at it. At the end of his third year of university, a school counsellor diagnosed Matt with mild obsessive tendencies. He was unable to complete his assignments on time, unsure as to whether he had done a perfect job. Despite these struggles, Matt graduated with top marks and became a highly functioning IT worker.

Shortly after establishing his career, he met Jane, a strong-minded woman of Korean descent, who was tolerant of Matt's obsessive way of coping with life. However, this equilibrium changed once Jane became ill with high levels of anxiety after the birth of their first child. She needed psychiatric intervention and was no longer emotionally available to him. Matt's obsessive thinking escalated rapidly. He began to have horrific,

(continued)

© Springer International Publishing AG 2018
S.K. Misri, *Paternal Postnatal Psychiatric Illnesses*,
https://doi.org/10.1007/978-3-319-68249-5_5

irrational thoughts, egodystonic in nature, about harming not only his newborn son but also his wife. He was especially petrified about handling knives and was afraid that he might actually stab the infant inadvertently. These intrusive thoughts began to affect profoundly; he lost sleep and became agitated. He became very anxious and finally presented to the emergency room, afraid he was "going crazy".

He was assessed by a psychiatrist, who eventually referred him to an OCD clinic where he started cognitive behaviour therapy. Three months into the treatment, his obsessive thoughts slowly became better, and he was able to function well. About 9 months after the baby's birth, it appeared that Matt's obsessions had cleared up and he was back to his baseline level of functioning, very different from the immediate postpartum period where he was highly incapacitated.

Matt's story is not unusual. Many first-time fathers after the birth of their babies do have fears around childbirth. They become obsessed with wanting to do the best for their newborn. For those struggling with these perfectionist tendencies, such as Matt, wanting to be a good provider and father becomes the ultimate dread; Matt responded to this fear with obsessions and very compulsions. In the case of Matt, the horrific, irrational thoughts were of sudden onset. He did not see them coming and responded to them with a great deal of fear. A compounding problem was that his wife was also psychiatrically ill and was not available for him to confide in. He suffered for the longest time, alone and internalizing his fears. The disturbing thoughts and images of him harming the baby and his partner were horrifying. This was a planned pregnancy, and they had waited for this baby for a while; the development of these intrusive thoughts towards his healthy newborn led to Matt's very high levels of anxiety. Eventually, with treatment, he learned to

(continued)

not avoid his baby, as one of the early manifestations of his illness was not wanting to be around knives when the baby was in the same room. The complicating factor was the presence of disturbing thoughts towards his spouse as well. There was a lot of guilt attached to having these thoughts, as Matt felt he was angry and upset that his wife was psychiatrically ill. When the thoughts began to pre-occupy his mind to a heightened degree, Matt became concerned that losing control and actually hurting his child might become a terrible consequence of his mental state. Therefore, getting help in time did alleviate the obsessive features. The compulsive behaviours fortunately had not escalated. He also needed further therapy with supportive counselling with regard to dealing with his feelings of guilt over not being a good father and incorporating the obsessional thoughts with cognitive restructuring.

DSM-5 Diagnosis

Obsessive-Compulsive Disorder

A. *Either obsessions or compulsions:*
   Obsessions as defined by (1), (2), (3) and (4):
1. *Recurrent and persistent thoughts, impulses or images that are experienced, at some time during the disturbance, as intrusive and inappropriate and that cause marked anxiety or distress.*
2. *The thoughts, impulses or images are not simply excessive worries about real-life problems.*
3. *The person attempts to ignore or suppress such thoughts, impulses or images or to neutralize them with some other thought or action.*

4. *The person recognizes that the obsessional thoughts, impulses or images are a product of his or her own mind (not imposed from without as in thought insertion) .*

Compulsions as defined by (1) and (2):

1. *Repetitive behaviours (e.g. handwashing, ordering, checking) or mental acts (e.g. praying, counting, repeating words silently) that the person feels driven to perform in response to an obsession, or according to rules that must be applied rigidly.*
2. *The behaviours or mental acts are aimed at preventing or reducing distress or preventing some dreaded event or situation; however, these behaviours or mental acts either are not connected in a realistic way with what they are designed to neutralize or prevent or are clearly excessive.*

B. *At some point during the course of the disorder, the person has recognized that the obsessions or compulsions are excessive or unreasonable.*
C. *The obsessions or compulsions cause marked distress, are time consuming (take more than 1 h a day) or significantly interfere with the person's normal routine, occupational (or academic) functioning or usual social activities or relationships.*
D. *If another Axis 1 disorder is present, the content of the obsessions or compulsions is not restricted to it (e.g. preoccupation with food in the presence of an eating disorder, hair pulling in the presence of trichotillomania with appearance in the presence of body dysmorphic disorder, preoccupation with drugs in the presence of a substance use disorder, preoccupation with having a serious illness in the presence of hypochondriasis, preoccupation with sexual urges or fantasies in the presence of a paraphilia or guilty ruminations in the presence of major depressive disorder).*
E. *The disturbance is not due to the direct physiological effects of a substance (e.g. a drug of abuse, a medication) or a general medical condition.*

Review of the Disorder

Introduction

In the early 2000s, Dr. Jonathan Abramowitz, a psychologist from the Mayo Clinic, was the first clinician to report four cases of paternal postpartum OCD. Obsessive-compulsive disorder during pregnancy or in the postpartum period in women has been previously reported with the most common occurrence of egodystonic intrusive thoughts that suddenly start to preoccupy a new mother's mind. These thoughts are extraordinarily anxiety-provoking and usually result in a great deal of impairment in most domains of a woman's life. The aetiology of such a disorder in the past was assigned to hormonal changes that occur either during pregnancy or in the postpartum period. The "serotonin hypothesis" suggested that the fluctuating levels of oestrogen and progesterone influenced the levels of serotonin which explained the onset of OCD. Therefore, OCD was earlier thought to be caused by serotonin dysfunction. As a result, little attention was paid to the occurrence of disturbing thoughts in males who do not go through the same hormonal fluctuations when their partner is either pregnant or postpartum. Rachman and colleagues suggested that obsessive-compulsive disorder is based on the understanding that most adults experience upsetting thoughts at some point. Some individuals respond to these thoughts in an unusual way by thinking that they may act upon them. This then becomes an increasingly pervasive fear and occupies their minds and controls their thoughts. Therefore, people with obsessional thoughts want to distract themselves by getting into compulsive rituals so that they can avoid thinking about these obsessive thoughts which are potentially threatening.

If one examines this model, then it is not difficult to understand that the birth of a vulnerable infant may evoke the development of obsessional thoughts about being responsible for this baby and increasing concern about the baby's welfare and the ability to protect the baby. Rachman and colleagues also went on to differentiate between normal obsessions and the associated distress with these thoughts. They further went on to note that such thoughts are often triggered by external stressors or stimuli. Studies now suggest that unwanted impulses can occur in the general population and are often precipitated by life circumstances. Therefore, the perinatal period presents as a vulnerable time, both for mother and father, who must accept a new level of responsibility in his adult life.

Studies thus far show that postpartum females are at a higher risk of developing OCD symptoms. The common obsessional thoughts that preoccupy a woman, especially after childbirth, include obsessional thoughts about harm coming to their infant. This could happen in a variety of ways. She could potentially stab the baby inadvertently, she could push the baby stroller into an oncoming car, she might also accidently drown the baby while bathing and/or suffocating the baby while putting the baby to bed, etc. These irrational thoughts are very disturbing and can be associated at times with depressive illness. Abramowitz and colleagues designed a study to assess the presence and phenomenology of postpartum obsessive-like intrusive thoughts and images, as well as impulses, in a large sample of parents with young infants. A survey was mailed to 300 child-bearing women and their partners who were biological fathers of the infants. The authors compiled a list of unwanted, upsetting, intrusive thoughts and divided them into seven categories. The seven categories included:

(a) Thoughts of suffocation or infant death syndrome
(b) Thoughts of accidents
(c) Unwanted urges of intentional harm
(d) Thoughts of losing the infant
(e) Illness
(f) Unexpected sexual thoughts
(g) Contamination

Both mothers and fathers were found to have intrusive thoughts; however, more mothers reported feeling distress from these thoughts compared to fathers. With regard to the fathers, the more difficulty they had in controlling these thoughts, the less comfortable they felt about disclosing these thoughts during the survey. Results of this study showed that intrusive and acceptable thoughts about infants are common, both in mothers and fathers of newborns, and that, although these are present in healthy parents, they sometimes resemble clinical obsessions as seen in patients with OCD. The fact that fathers also have these intrusive thoughts suggests that other factors need to be examined with regard to development of these obsessional thoughts. Stress appears to be one factor that could explain why fathers revert to having these threatening ruminations about their children. The question remains whether these healthy individuals who experience these unwanted thoughts are at a greater risk for developing full-fledged OCD symptoms. Another possibility is that these normal, unwanted, upsetting thoughts and the clinical manifestation of OCD may be on a continuum.

Epidemiology

The exact incidence or prevalence of postpartum OCD is unknown. The lifetime prevalence rate of OCD in the general population is about 2–3% and is consistent across different cultures. However, what is clear is that lifetime prevalence of OCD may be slightly higher in women compared to men at 3.1% versus 2%. Some studies suggest that the incidence of OCD in women is highest during child-bearing years.

Prevalence Rates and Diagnosis of Postpartum Depression in Fathers

In a study by Coelho, the researchers attempted to describe the prevalence rates and correlates of OCD in Brazilian fathers in the third trimester of pregnancy and in the first 2 months postpartum. They administered a variety of different measures to 707 fathers, which included the MINI at 28–34 weeks of pregnancy and 30–60 days postpartum.

Interesting results were obtained from the fathers: the prevalence rate of OCD was found to be 3.4% in the third trimester of pregnancy and 1.8% in the postpartum period. Most postpartum cases were new onset. They also found that OCD in fathers during pregnancy was associated with both unipolar and bipolar depression. Of note, OCD in fathers was significantly associated with OCD in mothers in both study periods, that is, in pregnancy and postpartum. This was the first study that investigated the prevalence, comorbid patterns and predictors of OCD in fathers during pregnancy and in the postpartum period. The study also showed that the comorbidity with bipolar spectrum disorder is frequent. OCD appears to be common in fathers both in pregnancy and postpartum. Therefore, the authors suggested that the partners of mothers who are diagnosed with OCD should also be evaluated.

The Course of OCD

The evidence available regarding the course of paternal OCD is very sparse at this point. With regard to perinatal OCD, it appears that the course of this illness is not very different from that seen in the general population. If it is not treated, the illness remains chronic and can fluctuate over a period of time. However, there is some difference between perinatal OCD and general OCD. Individuals who suffer from obsessional aggressive thoughts about harming the baby appear to have a better prognosis if treated early enough compared to individuals where compulsions are involved. Moreover, it is important to understand whether maternal or paternal postpartum OCD is a separate specific subtype of general OCD, and this will only be answered if the methodological issues that confuse the picture at this time are addressed. Not having proper definitions for OCD, both in fathers and mothers, makes it particularly difficult to address the question of whether or not this is a subtype. What is clear, however, is that perinatal OCD in women and men appears to present as a distinct clinical entity, whereas episodes of depression which occur in new parents are not indistinguishable from those occurring at other times. Intrusive, upsetting, ego-dystonic thoughts are reflective of a person's concerns about changes in their life after the birth of a baby. Nonetheless, more research is needed, both clinically and in non-clinical populations to indicate whether only a select few experience these highly disturbing thoughts.

There is also the added pressure on fathers and mothers today with regard to what the "perfect parenthood looks like". Therefore, not meeting these present societal norms can work negatively for the father, who may not ever match the image of confidence that is expected of him. One explanation could be that the ambivalence towards new father-hood may reflect the egodystonic thoughts of harming their infant because of their inability to deal with their emotions of fear and conflict, thus internalizing them through such thoughts. Because there are as yet no studies that directly compare whether these intrusive thoughts of a non-clinical sample eventually translate to manifestation of full-fledged OCD, we need to separate those who have a new-onset OCD from those who had a pre-existing OCD. By this process, we can identify whether these fathers and mothers too are at a higher risk later on for developing the disease. Health-care providers should be able to ask whether the father suffers from specific obsessions or compulsions and to also learn to differentiate between what is a normal intrusion versus what is not.

Comorbidity

Comorbid conditions of OCD, and major depressive disorder are most common in female patients. Sichel and colleagues described case reports of fifteen patients, nine of whom developed secondary major depression a few weeks after the onset of OCD. No systematic studies exist that describe comorbidity in fathers, although in clinical practice, many fathers report depressed mood with feelings of guilt and remorse when they have images of hurting their newborn. This new unexpected reality more often than not impacts their mood. In another study done by Williams and Koran in the 1990s, it was found that 9 out of the 24 patients with pre-existing OCD reported postpartum depression. In general population, the concurrent occurrence of depression, panic attacks and OCD is not uncommon. Comorbidity between OCD and anxiety is not infrequent.

It is important to differentiate between postpartum psychosis and postpartum OCD in new mothers as well as new fathers. There is no reference to postpartum psychosis in fathers in the literature. In women, postpartum psychosis is considered to be a manifestation of bipolar disease and is fortunately a rare condition which occurs in about one or two in a thousand postpartum women. In patients who suffer from OCD, their thoughts are egodystonic, whereas in those who suffer from psychosis, their thoughts are egosyntonic. In the case of postpartum psychosis, the person's delusional thinking and behaviour is associated with an increased risk of infanticide. Conversely, postpartum intrusive thoughts or obsessions are not associated with an increased risk of harming the baby. Instead, those with postpartum OCD try to deal with their thoughts by avoiding the situation that brings about the anxiety and try to resist their obsessional thoughts.

Fairbrother and colleagues suggest a cognitive behaviour model for postpartum OCD which should be able to account for the following:

1. Rapid onset of symptoms that occur in the perinatal period
2. The specificity of symptom presentation, i.e. harm coming to the infant as opposed to contamination or holding
3. The presence of symptoms in mothers and fathers of the newborn
4. That most parents of newborns experience intrusive, distressing thoughts related to their infants but relatively few go on to develop OCD symptoms

The authors go on to propose that the perinatal period lowers the threshold for OCD and sets the stage for misinterpretation of normally occurring intrusive infant-related thoughts to be threatening the development of behavioural patterns in response to intrusive thoughts. These may include, for instance, checking and rechecking the baby, avoiding the child, etc. It appears that first-time parents are probably more prone to experiencing postpartum OCD as compared to those who have had subsequent children. This is because the emotional impact of a second and third child arriving is typically much less significant than what is seen with the birth of the firstborn. One of the earliest studies about parenting was published in the late 1990s by Leckman and colleagues. The study focused on early parental preoccupation and behaviours surrounding the birth of a new family member. This was a longitudinal study at 8 months that included pregnant and postpartum mothers. They interviewed 41 pairs of parents. The hypothesis of this study was that the preoccupation about behaviours of the infant would peak for both parents close to birth of the child. A variety of measures were provided to the parents to record their behaviours. The study found that the parents of firstborn were more preoccupied and that higher caretaking responsibility was associated with higher preoccupation of both parents with regard to their infant, and 68% of the mothers and 76% of the fathers showed thoughts similar to OCD at 8 months. Up to 95% of the parents in this study reported at least one repetitive behaviour or thought; the findings showed that heightened sensitivity towards the baby may lead to maladaptive patterns of thinking. The conclusion of this study was that the symptoms resembling OCD can be found in postpartum parents who are preoccupied with their infant's behaviours more so than those who are not. While this study is not geared towards diagnosing OCD, either in mothers or fathers, it does give insight into the characteristics of parents who might be more vulnerable to the development of OCD.

Consequences for Infants and Children

Studies on children who have a parent suffering from mental illness have been done regarding certain types of psychiatric disorders, such as depression, addiction disorders, attention deficit disorders and anxiety disorders. It appears that there are currently very limited studies on children born to parents who have obsessive-compulsive disorder. What is available with regard to the children of parents who have OCD compared to those who do not is that these children generally have high rates of anxiety disorders, mood disorders and subclinical obsessive-compulsive disorders. Studies with regard to depression show that the illness in parents triggers an earlier onset of disorders in the children. In addition, the course of these disorders in children appears to be more protracted. Based on the present data, early treatment of mentally ill parents could benefit their children in the long run.

Black and colleagues in 2003 examined the association between parental OCD and emotional and behavioural disorders in their offspring. Their hypothesis was that the offspring of parents with OCD would show greater levels of anxiety, depression and obsessional symptoms than those seen in the controls. The researchers recruited 21 adults from the outpatient department of a hospital in Iowa who had a DSM-4 diagnosis of OCD and were in treatment for obsessive-compulsive disorder. Controls were matched for age and gender. Participants, as well as controls, had children between the ages of 7 and 18 years, and children were administered a variety of scales including the Child Behaviour Checklist (CBCL). The results of the study showed that children who had a parent with OCD had more pathological scores and they showed evidence of somatic complaints and displayed emotional and behavioural disturbances. They also had a higher incidence of anxiety disorders, panic disorder and social phobia. In addition, they were less likely to be employed and had lower income than those of the controls, although this finding was not statistically significant. As well, those with high CBCL scores were more likely to have parents with OCD. The conclusion of the study was that children whose parents have OCD are more likely than control offspring to have social, emotional and behavioural disorders.

The findings of this study raise very important questions with regard to how and why parents' illness affects their children. It is possible that in some children, the symptoms represent manifestation of early onset of OCD or another disorder within the OCD spectrum. This may have to do with genetically transmitted vulnerability from the parents. This is not different from earlier studies of depression and panic disorder where there was a link between emotional disturbances in the offspring and the presence of these illnesses in the parents. Another possibility could be that if the children are living in an environment where there is a parent who suffers from mental illness, they are watching the dysfunctional behaviour of this parent and are modelling themselves accordingly. It is also known that parents with OCD who have maladapted patterns of behaviour in their marriage sometimes may also involve their children in their ritualistic behaviours. Therefore, it is not only important to address the issues in the parents but also to watch out for the onset in the children. As yet, studies of the offspring where fathers alone suffer from OCD are non-existent, but clearly Black et al.'s study demonstrates the need to pay attention to not only the partners of mothers who suffer from OCD but also the children. Therefore, OCD is an illness that spares nobody. It is more prevalent in females than males; however, clinicians need to be aware of the possibility of the father suffering from this illness and also their offspring in the long run.

Recommendations: How Do You Intervene?

Screening and Diagnosis

It is important for the primary care physician, be it a family doctor, obstetrician or paediatrician, or for that matter a psychiatrist who sees postpartum women, to screen for symptoms of OCD in the father in the first few weeks, if not the first few months postpartum. It is not adequate to do one-time screening and come to a conclusion or a diagnosis of

OCD. It is important to follow these patients over a period of time to ascertain whether these unusual thoughts are a healthy response to a stressful situation like going through childbirth or if they are indicative of impending OCD. Enquiries should also be made about the compulsive checking behaviours and past history of OCD as a child and if these disorders exist in family members. These are all additional risk factors that make a person vulnerable in the postpartum period. Sometimes, administering the Y-BOCS could also be used to evaluate the severity of symptoms, in addition to monitoring response to the treatment. Detailed enquiry with regard to the frequency and intensity of thoughts should also be considered. In addition, thorough examination and assessment of psychiatric symptoms are warranted, because there may be comorbidity with other psychiatric disorders such as generalized anxiety disorder and/or depression. There is a difference between obsessions related to ruminations associated with major depression and those that occur de novo and are egodystonic, intrusive thoughts about harm coming to the infant. When excessive worry or anxiety is present, which interferes with functioning, a detailed examination of generalized anxiety symptoms is recommended.

Treatment

There are a variety of different treatments available for managing the symptoms of obsessive-compulsive disorders. Cognitive behaviour therapy by exposure and response prevention, or ERP, is now considered the best possible available psychotherapy for OCD. Pharmacotherapy with a variety of selective serotonin reuptake inhibitors has also been tried. These include sertraline, paroxetine, fluoxetine, citalopram and fluvoxamine. Both psychotherapy and pharmacotherapy have been shown to be efficacious treatments. There is a small percentage of patents in general population that remain resistant to treatment and not all benefit from these interventions; many patients remain symptomatic with OCD for a long duration.

Dr. Edna Foa conducted a randomized placebo-controlled trial of exposure and ritual prevention, with clomipramine alone, and combination of these two in treating obsessive-compulsive disorder. One hundred and twenty-two participants were enrolled and randomized to either a placebo-controlled trial of exposure and ritual prevention, clomipramine alone and a combination of both and a placebo. Participant outcome was measured by the Yale-Brown Obsessive-Compulsive Scale or Y-BOCS. Results at 12 weeks showed that all treatment groups improved compared to the placebo group and that exposure and ritual prevention appeared to be more effective than clomipramine. The researchers also found that the combined treatment was better than clomipramine alone but not superior to exposure and ritual prevention treatment alone. The conclusion of the study was that the ERP seemed to have high efficacy compared to clomipramine but the combined treatment was useful where ERP was not intensively conducted. Earlier findings of whether or not ERP is superior to pharmacotherapy showed that there is inconsistency in the outcome. The outcome seems to depend on the frequency of the ERP treatment, e.g. daily exposure versus weekly exposure. Also, the affordability of such treatment is an interesting point. Not everyone can afford ERP treatment, putting this type of treatment out of reach for them. So although this study was encouraging with regard to the efficacy of ERP, it is not widely available. Conversely, SSRI medications are easily available, they have less time commitment, and people tend to be more able to access pharmacotherapy versus psychotherapy in most countries.

There is no data as yet with regard to treatments that are specifically conducted in postpartum fathers who suffer from OCD. It appears that methods that are used to treat OCD in the general population would be effective in fathers as well. The effectiveness of ERP has been accepted widely. However, the differential effectiveness of behavioural and cognitive approaches has shown inconclusive results. A meta-analysis on the effectiveness of psychological treatment of OCD identified 19 studies which met the selection criteria as set out by Rosa-Alcazar and her colleagues. The researchers found that the therapist-guided exposure was better than therapist-assisted self-exposure, and exposure in vivo combined with exposure in imagination was better than exposure in vivo alone. Their conclusion was that ERP and cognitive restructuring were both effective in treating OCD, but there was no advantage using them in a combined fashion. The researchers also found that if there was a comorbid presence of other psychiatric disorders such as depression or anxiety disorders, these patients did not do well with either ERP or ERP and cognitive restructuring.

Group treatment seems to have achieved similar results to individual therapy in this particular research, which is encouraging, as this might help reduce cost and also the resources necessary to implement such treatment. To date, no CBT trials in postpartum populations have been implemented. Trials of exposure and response prevention in patients with obsessional thoughts without compulsions, which are frequently seen in the perinatal population, have produced inconsistent results. It is important to ascertain whether the postpartum fathers are avoiding contact with their infants or are seeking assurances from the other health-care providers and/or are busy with mental rituals, because these may be similar to overt compulsions and may be more amenable to treatment with CBT. For those fathers who have intrusive obsessional thoughts without compulsions, pharmacotherapy may be an effective option. This kind of treatment has been found to be effective in the treatment of OCD in the general population. In a case study done by Sichel and colleagues, 15 patients were treated with SSRIs such as fluoxetine, clomipramine and desipramine. The researchers found that patients did well up to about 1 year postpartum. Some of the patients remained on pharmacotherapy because of the presence of residual symptoms. In clinical practice, it is not unusual to see high SSRI dosage levels used to treat OCD compared to other illnesses such as depression. It appears that the therapeutic response to treat OCD occurs at a higher dose. It is important to treat fathers with OCD with psychotherapy, pharmaco-therapy or a combination wherever it is available, in order to avoid marital disruption. The expectant father, as well as their health-care professional, should be educated about the symptoms of postpartum OCD in fathers. Identifying the risk factors is important to minimize short- and long-term effects.

Take-Home Messages

1. Pregnancy and the postpartum period present a time of high vulnerability for development of obsessional problems in both males and females.
2. The cognitive behaviour model of OCD suggests that most adults normally experience intrusive, upsetting, egodystonic thoughts. It is when the individuals find these benign thoughts to be threatening that the possibility of greater frequency of such thoughts increases, resulting in OCD.
3. It is likely that normal, unwanted intrusive thoughts are at one end of the spectrum, while OCD happens to be at the other end of the spectrum, especially for postpartum fathers.
4. This theory is in opposition to the neurobiological model of OCD which assigns serotonin system dysfunction as an etiological factor in the development of OCD.
5. Repeated upsetting thoughts of harming the infant are egodystonic and occur in both males and females, while egosyntonic intrusive thoughts occur in postpartum psychosis.
6. Treatment consists of cognitive behaviour therapy with ERP and cognitive restructuring and psychoeducation. Pharmacotherapy with SSRIs as well as SNRIs is also effective.

References

1. Andreasen NC. What is post-traumatic stress disorder? Dialogues Clin Neurosci. 2011;13(3):240.
2. Berger W, Coutinho ES, Figueira I, et al. Rescuers at risk: a systematic review and meta-regression analysis of the worldwide

current prevalence and correlates of PTSD in rescue workers. Soc Psychiatry Psychiatr Epidemiol. 2012;47(6):1001–11.

3. Borghini A, Habersaat S, Forcada-Guex M, et al. Effects of an early intervention on maternal post-traumatic stress symptoms and the quality of mother–infant interaction: the case of preterm birth. Infant Behav Dev. 2014;37(4):624–31.

4. Crocq MA, Crocq L. From shell shock and war neurosis to posttraumatic stress disorder: a history of psychotraumatology. Dialogues Clin Neurosci. 2000;2(1):47–55.

5. Di Blasio P, Ionio C. Postpartum stress symptoms and child temperament: a follow-up study. J Prenat Perinat Psychol Health. 2005;19(3):185–98.

6. Feeley N, Zelkowitz P, Cormier C, et al. Posttraumatic stress among mothers of very low birthweight infants at 6 months after discharge from the neonatal intensive care unit. Appl Nurs Res. 2011;24(2):114–7.

7. Frans Ö, Rimmö PA, Åberg L, et al. Trauma exposure and post-traumatic stress disorder in the general population. Acta Psychiatr Scand. 2005;111(4):291–300.

8. Friedman MJ, Bernardy NC. Considering future pharmacotherapy for PTSD. Neurosci Lett. 2016;649:181.

9. Galovski T, Lyons JA. Psychological sequelae of combat violence: a review of the impact of PTSD on the veteran's family and possible interventions. Aggress Violent Behav. 2004;9(5):477–501.

10. Jones E, Fear D, Phil NT, et al. Shell shock and mild traumatic brain injury: a historical review. Am J Psychiatry. 2007;164(11):1641–5.

11. Kar N. Cognitive behavioral therapy for the treatment of posttraumatic stress disorder: a review. Neuropsychiatr Dis Treat. 2011;7(1):167–81.

12. Olde E, van der Hart O, Kleber R, et al. Posttraumatic stress following childbirth: a review. Clin Psychol Rev. 2006;26(1):1–6.

13. Onoye JM, Shafer LA, Goebert DA, et al. Changes in PTSD symptomatology and mental health during pregnancy and postpartum. Arch Womens Ment Health. 2013;16(6):453–63.

14. Pierrehumbert B, Nicole A, Muller-Nix C, et al. Parental posttraumatic reactions after premature birth: implications for sleeping and eating problems in the infant. Arch Dis Child Fetal Neonatal Ed. 2003;88(5):400–4.

15. Resick PA, Wachen JS, Dondanville KA, et al. Effect of group vs individual cognitive processing therapy in active-duty military seeking treatment for posttraumatic stress disorder: a randomized clinical trial. JAMA Psychiat. 2017;74(1):28–36.

16. Santiago PN, Ursano RJ, Gray CL, et al. A systematic review of PTSD prevalence and trajectories in DSM-5 defined trauma exposed populations: intentional and non-intentional traumatic events. PLoS One. 2013;8(4):e59236.

17. Sayer NA, Friedemann-Sanchez G, Spoont M, et al. A qualitative study of determinants of PTSD treatment initiation in veterans. Psychiatry. 2009;72(3):238–55.

18. Schlenger WE, Mulvaney-Day N, Williams CS, et al. PTSD and use of outpatient general medical services among veterans of the Vietnam war. Psych Serv. 2016;67(5):543–50.

19. Shaw RJ, Bernard RS, DeBlois T, et al. The relationship between acute stress disorder and posttraumatic stress disorder in the neonatal intensive care unit. Psychosomatics. 2009;50(2):131–7.

20. Smith TC, Wingard DL, Ryan MA, et al. PTSD prevalence, associated exposures, and functional health outcomes in a large, population-based military cohort. Public Health Rep. 2009;124(1):90–102.

21. Solomon SD, Johnson DM. Psychosocial treatment of post-traumatic stress disorder: a practice-friendly review of outcome research. J Clin Psychol. 2002;58(8):947–59.

22. Stein DJ, Ipser J, McAnda N. Pharmacotherapy of posttraumatic stress disorder: a review of meta-analyses and treatment guidelines. CNS Spectr. 2009;14(1):25–31.

23. Taylor S, Thordarson DS, Maxfield L, et al. Comparative efficacy, speed, and adverse effects of three PTSD treatments: exposure therapy, EMDR, and relaxation training. J Consult Clin Psychol. 2003;71(2):330.

24. Van Ameringen M, Mancini C, Patterson B, et al. Post-traumatic stress disorder in Canada. CNS Neurosci Ther. 2008;14(3):171–81.

Chapter 6
Marital Discord and Childbirth: Increasing Conflicts in New Parents

Dad's Story: Clinical Vignette

Rico, a 39-year-old carpenter, well known for his expertise in finishing work in heritage homes, was an outgoing man who made friends easily. He was kind, considerate and involved in his community. His parents came as refugees from Central America, something that Rico was very proud of. He married his childhood sweetheart, Melissa, with whom he went to school. Their parents were neighbours and knew each other very well. Within the first year of their marriage, Melissa found it particularly strenuous to balance the pressures of her demanding job as a social worker and running a household. She received little help from Rico, whose work schedule was often unpredictable, thereby increasing Melissa's domestic responsibilities. She knew that maintaining the household was expected of her, as Rico grew up in a family where keeping a tidy home and cooking sumptuous meals were valued. During pregnancy, Melissa became increasingly despondent over her lack of support from Rico, her ongoing isolation and his decreased emotional involvement in the pregnancy. After the birth of Susie, their relationship discord escalated with increasing con-

(continued)

© Springer International Publishing AG 2018
S.K. Misri, *Paternal Postnatal Psychiatric Illnesses*,
https://doi.org/10.1007/978-3-319-68249-5_6

flict, the inability to resolve differences amicably, irritability and hostility. Lack of sleep and mounting frustration further impeded their transition to parenthood. When Susie turned 2 years of age, Melissa realized that the only way to salvage her relationship with Rico was to seek marital therapy. With her background as a social worker, she was aware that unless the interpersonal conflict and their individual behaviours changed, a long-term negative impact on Susie would be inevitable. Rico grew up witnessing his mother's accommodating, non-assertive and at times passive behaviours in response to his father's short temper and verbal abuse. In therapy, Rico admitted that he expected Melissa to behave not dissimilarly to his mother. It took him time to understand his denial and his own role in perpetuating their marital conflict.

Melissa and Rico appeared outwardly to be a "perfect match". However, they came from two very different backgrounds. It is not uncommon for one partner in a relationship to exhibit behaviours that they were familiar with while growing up with their own family of origin. Rico's parents came as refugees from Central America and had a very rough time adjusting to a new country but became quite successful with his father's work as a construction contractor. Rico went to a carpentry trade school and became highly specialized in his skill and took pride in his work. He grew up in a traditional household, where his mother looked after all the needs of the men at home, and there were several, as Rico was one of four siblings, all brothers. Rico and his brothers were not expected to help out in the household. Consequently, he watched his mother take responsibility for running the entire household in an efficient manner. However, there were many scary and fearful moments in his life, which he never really dealt with or wanted to come to terms with. One was his father's unpredictable temper tantrums and the uncertainty of when they might occur, as well as the way

(continued)

in which his mother dealt with the occasionally resulting abuse. To him, this was "normal". He did not know anything different. Somehow in his mind, this behaviour pattern between his parents was acceptable. Melissa, who came from a completely different type of background with both parents working, brought into the marriage a sense of equality and an expectation that there would be mutual respect over the passage of time. She was not accustomed to emotional outbursts or loud arguments and could not deal with the way in which Rico dealt with conflict. Over time, she became withdrawn, became more involved in her work and at the same time started to resent where their relationship was going. After the baby's birth, this couple grew apart considerably. They were no longer civil to one another, and very soon it became obvious, especially to Melissa, that the relationship was on shaky ground. Most of all, she was concerned about the impact on little Susie, who was now also having temper tantrums. Susie was difficult to console and was showing oppositional behaviours. This caused a lot of anxiety in Melissa, who finally decided to seek therapy for the two of them. Both Melissa and Rico had many different behavioural patterns and reasons why they would blame one another, and these became evident in therapy. The couple made a concerted effort to cope with their stormy relationship in a positive manner and especially to give Susie a good life within an "intact family".

DSM-5 Diagnosis

1. *Relationship Distress with Spouse or Intimate Partner. This category should be used when the major focus of the clinical contact is to address the quality of the intimate (spouse or partner) relationship or when the quality of their relationship is affecting the course, prognosis or treatment of a mental or other medical disorders. Partners can be of*

the same or different genders. Typically, their relationship distress is associated with impaired functioning in behaviour, cognitive or affective domains. Examples of behaviour problems include conflict resolution difficulty, withdrawal and other over-involvement. Cognitive problems can manifest as chronic negative attributions of the other's intensions or dismissals of partner's positive behaviours. Affective problems would include chronic sadness, apathy and/or anger about the other partner.

2. *Phase of Life Problem. This category should be used when a problem adjusting to a life cycle transition (a particular developmental phase is the focus of clinical attention) has an impact on the individual's treatment or prognosis. Examples of such transitions include entering or completing school, leaving parental control, getting married, starting a new career, becoming a parent, adjusting to emptiness after children leave home and retiring.*

Review of the Disorder

Epidemiology

The birth of the first baby often impacts the quality of the marital relationship for both parents. Interpersonal relationships change, which requires adjustment to the new situation of becoming parents in addition to the challenges that new parenthood brings. Generally, the experiences with the family of origin are brought into the relationship by each parent, impacting marital quality. In a study of the intergenerational transmission of marital quality during the transition to parenthood, Parren and colleagues aimed to investigate the impact of the quality of the family of origin's marriage on marital quality after the birth of a child. The researchers conducted a longitudinal study where questionnaires were administered to participants during pregnancy and 12 months after the birth of their first child. A total of 62 first-time parents completed self-reported marital satisfaction questionnaires and were also interviewed to evaluate the quality of the couple's dialogue. The results showed that couples with negative recollection of their family of origin marriages showed more negative changes. Overall, the study showed that husbands' and wives' recollection of their family of origin marriage predicted the changes in their marital quality. Specifically, fathers with a high-quality family of origin marriage had higher overall marital satisfaction and a better communication pattern. Similarly, mothers who recollected positive family of origin marriages reported no increases in conflict. It was unclear whether these associations were due to real experiences within one's family of origin or to mental recollections or even the current role of the young parents. Several different factors have been proposed to explain this intergenerational transmission of negative marital quality and/or divorce. Social learning patterns play a strong role, and modelling oneself after their parents' marriage is another factor. Increased stressful experiences during transitioning to parenthood are an important consideration which may explain some of the difficulties a young couple may experience as they embark on parenthood. It is also possible that the actual roles that some of the grandparents are able to play in the life of their new family may affect the course of the parental partnership. This was partly true in the case of Melissa and Rico, as Rico's parents continued to be actively involved in the raising of Susie. Melissa was afraid that a similar pattern would evolve in her own marriage, that is, that Rico would continue to expect non-assertive behaviour. In addition, Melissa was worried that her little girl may be affected by such an environment that persisted in Rico's parents' household. She wanted to break away from that pattern of parental relationship.

Another issue in the raising of Susie, both for Rico and Melissa, was understanding Rico's role as a new father in this triadic relationship. Research on fathers' involvement with newborn babies and children has been evolving for the past few decades. Many factors impact paternal involvement generally in the day-to-day caring of the children, such as their perceived sense of responsibility and balancing this with stresses at work and at home. In a marriage which is stable, generally, involvement of the father is seen in a positive light. Many studies have examined how marital satisfaction is related to father involvement. Mixed findings have been reported. While some studies have found that there is a relationship between marital satisfaction and father's involvement, others have found that there is no correlation. What is clear, however, is that transitioning to parenthood is an important phase of life and is clearly going to have a differential impact on both parents, as was the case with Melissa and Rico. Moving away from traditional roles within the family for Rico was much more difficult than it was for Melissa. In a longitudinal study done by Lee and Doherty, marital satisfaction and father involvement during the transition to parenthood were examined. Their study consisted of self-reports, time diaries and in-home observation of parent-child interactions. The data was collected from 165 couples during the second trimester of pregnancy and 6 and 12 months postpartum. Results of the study showed that the more satisfied a father felt in the marriage before birth, the more time he spent with the child. Higher quality of involvement led to more emotional support, more father-child dyadic synchrony, more warmth in their relationship and less intrusiveness. The researchers found that a decrease in the father's marital satisfaction from the second trimester to 6 months postpartum led to decreasing quality of involvement with their own children. In addition, attitude about fathering also played an important role when young men became fathers. For instance, when the new fathers have a positive attitude towards being involved with their children, then one would expect that they would be likely a part of their children's lives. However, marital satisfaction may play an important role in changing such a relationship. Therefore, it is important to know how the mother feels towards the father's involvement with the child as well. For instance, if the mother's attitude towards father's involvement is positive, one may expect a positive relationship between father's marital satisfaction and involvement with their children because a satisfying marital relationship may motivate fathers to get more involved. Another finding that was interesting in this particular research was the father's attitude towards working mothers. For instance, in this study, the results showed that when mothers worked for more hours per week, father's prenatal marital satisfaction had a positive influence on the total quantity of paternal involvement. On the other hand, if the mother worked less outside of the home, this relationship was negative. So it appears that the mother's employment and father's attitude towards involvement with their children are additional moderators towards marital satisfaction. Given the complexity of the association between marital satisfaction, father involvement and maternal work issues, it appears that there is clearly a relationship between all these factors. However, more studies in the future are required to further confirm these findings, as the literature in the past has been conflicting, or mixed, with regard to the findings of this particular study.

Marriage and Psychiatric Disorders in Partners

A high rate of depression and marital discord has been addressed in the literature. In a 2-year prospective longitudinal study, Wisman and Uebelacker looked at the associations between marital discord and depressive symptoms in middle-aged adults. The study surveyed 1869 couples over the course of 2 years, which involved administering personal interviews and questionnaires to the participants. Two waves of data were collected from 2002 to 2003 and from 2004 to 2005. Appropriate questionnaires were included to measure depression as well as marital discord. The researchers found that baseline marital discord was significantly associated with depressive symptoms and baseline depressive symptoms were significantly associated with follow-up marital discord, both for husbands and wives. In other words, no gender differences were found within couples. The study concluded that there may be a bidirectional longitudinal association between marital discord and depressive symptoms in middle- and older-aged adults. It is important to note that these individuals were experiencing depressive symptoms but were not diagnosed with depression. This study goes to show that depressive symptoms in one person can predict changes in the spouse's marital relationship. In clinical practice, it is not uncommon to see how postpartum depression in new mothers impacts the trajectory of an otherwise stable relationship. Depressive illness can have varied effects on interpersonal behaviours towards the partner. It can cause interruption in intimacy between partners as well as compromising the maternal role. All these factors generally create a substantial amount of stress for the young couple. In modern marriages, the husband may occasionally be at a loss as to how to deal with increasing demands of daily life as a new father as well as how to deal with a wife who is suffering from depression. Similarly, a mother who is living with a partner who suffers from ongoing psychiatric illness has a difficult time maintaining harmony within the relationship. Therefore, relationship discord can either predate psychiatric disorder onset or predict depressive symptoms. This was again addressed by Wisman in 2012 where an association was reviewed between poor relationship adjustment and/or discord and the prevalence, incidence and treatment of psychopathology. A review of the literature showed that relationship discord is more strongly associated with men who have lower self-esteem and people with higher levels of anxious-ambivalent attachment and blame-oriented attributions about partners' negative behaviours. In therapy, over time, Rico learned that underneath this façade of being a successful finishing carpenter, his self-esteem was low, and he felt competitive with his highly accomplished wife, having a very ambivalent attachment in general to females.

Whisman's 2012 study also showed that those with a genetic predisposition to internalizing psychopathology may be more likely to experience internalizing symptoms if they were in a discordant relationship. Therefore, it appears that there is an association between relationship discord and depressive symptoms, especially for those who suffer from chronic dysphoria, women in poverty, those with high levels of neuroticism and women with low levels of masculinity. People in discordant relationships also may be less likely to respond to individually based treatment. It is important to treat the relationship first before any individual treatment is undertaken. It also appears that there is an increase in the likelihood of relapse of marital dysfunction after pharmaco-therapy and/or psychotherapy in those individuals who are chronically depressed. Poor marital adjustment has been shown to predict increased likelihood of relapse for those with substance use issues as well. It is important therefore for clinicians to understand that treatment focused on improving relationship functioning is an integral part of treating psychiatric disorders in partners.

In addition to depression, bipolar illness, alcohol abuse and generalized anxiety disorder are also associated with a high level of marital distress. Interestingly enough, panic disorder seems to be the only exception with regard to anxiety symptoms. The conclusion of this study examining marital distress and Axis 1 DSM diagnoses showed that there is a strong correlation between couples' functioning and mental health/psychiatric disorders.

Sleep Disruption and Decline in Marital Satisfaction

Lack of sleep in new mothers is a constant source of frustration when transitioning to parenthood. If the baby is difficult to soothe or if there are nursing issues that arise in the first few weeks, the lack of sleep and the anxiety associated with the baby's development can place an extraordinary burden on a young couple. It is not uncommon for working fathers to be separated in a different room or to sleep on the couch, while the mother is up all night tending to the baby's needs. This can create distance between the couple, reduce their communication and increase the sense of isolation for a young mother, who is trying to deal with the baby almost exclusively. However, although these parental dynamics are changing in modern times, they have not yet completely evolved. For the first few months when a mother is breast-feeding the baby, sleep disruption is inevitable. Common issues that arise as a result of sleep deprivation include blaming one another in the marriage, angry outbursts, increased irritability, exhaustion, fatigue and a lack of concentration. Often, chronic sleep deprivation is linked to negative mood and at times can be a trigger for depressive illness. Increased marital conflict, decreased positive spousal interaction, feelings of chaos and disappointment can herald the transition to parenthood. The contribution of sleep disruption is significant in this specific phase of life when both the parents are trying to figure out the new roles assigned to them. Despite this well-documented consequence of sleep deprivation, mood and cognition, it seems that studies are sparse in confirming such a relationship in a conclusive manner. In a study by Medina and colleagues, the researchers used the terms "sleep disturbance" and "sleep disruption" interchangeably to examine how these conditions can diminish marital satisfaction. The sleep of new parents is often disturbed for weeks on end, and this can have a deleterious effect on the wellness of both partners. This study showed that new mothers experience a greater sleep disturbance after the birth of a child in the postpartum period and that better quality of sleep may act as a buffer. Additionally, sleep deprivation was associated with extra-punitive and blaming responses to frustrating situations. This study showed that the transition to parenthood led to a significant increase in conflict and a decrease in positive marital interaction. Therefore, the authors concluded that sleep disruption has an important contributory role in marital satisfaction and that it is important for health-care providers to enquire about insomnia or sleep disturbance. This should be an important aspect of the overall assessment of postpartum depression and/or marital stability, and an in-depth enquiry about roles assigned to care for the baby at night should be included. For instance, it is not unusual for a sleep-deprived mother to hand over a bottle to her partner and/or have a sleep schedule whereby each partner wakes up at a certain time in order to deal with this very difficult, but realistic, issue that young couples face.

The Effects of Marital Dysfunction on the Children

It is not unusual to encounter differences between parents with regard to how they wish to raise their children. Interpersonal differences have to be respected and must be dealt with in a mature manner in order to not negatively impact the child and later on the adolescent. Different modes of conflict expression and resolution, which include avoidant, overt or covert conflicting styles, appear to be the mode of expression when parenting styles are involved. This particular issue was reviewed by Krishnakumar and Buehler. In this study, they wanted to build on earlier models of association between global marital quality and parent-child relations. They reviewed 39 publications from 1981 to 1998 that examined the association between interpersonal conflict and parenting behaviours. The results of the review showed that there is a general negative relationship between interpersonal conflicts and parenting behaviours where parental preoccupation with marital conflict impairs most dimensions of child-rearing. The strongest negative impact was seen in harsh discipline and lower levels of parental acceptance. The review findings support the spillover hypothesis where the emotions and tensions aroused during negative marital interactions are carried over into parent-child interactions. The study also found that marital hostility and aggressions are more strongly associated with parenting quality in married families than divorced families. Thirdly, the association between interpersonal conflict and quality of parenting was stronger for girls, suggesting that parents who are aggressive in their relationship are more hostile and negative towards their daughters as compared to their sons. The conclusion of this study was that there is a moderate association between inter-parental conflict and parenting behaviours, with the strongest impact on children being harsh discipline and low levels of parental acceptance. This study also shows that there is little support for the notion that parents can compartmentalize their marital distress from their roles as parents. These two issues are intimately connected. Therefore, the importance of having a stable marital relationship prior to conception and/or having a child cannot be overstated. As was evident with Rico and Melissa, some of the interpersonal issues on which they disagreed were present prior to her becoming pregnant and only escalated after the birth of Susie. This is not an uncommon occurrence in many couples and is further confirmed by studies such as Krishnakumar and Buehler's. The spillover hypothesis proposes that emotions and tensions within the marriage can spill over, or be carried into, parent-child interaction. This interpretation is consistent with the findings of the subject study. This area of research is important in that it will help families to get help when needed by seeking early intervention so as to prevent short- and long-term impacts on their growing children, as well as learn positive ways of dealing with their conflicts in the presence of their children.

The children's emotional and behavioural functioning is linked to interpersonal conflict of their parents. However, not all children who witness such behaviours necessarily show dysfunction. A meta-analysis conducted by Kimberly Rhoades in 2008 focused on children's responses to conflicts. The author felt that children's own responses to interpersonal conflicts are most proximal to their psychosocial and physical adjustment and that these responses may provide an index of how children interpret and cope with interpersonal conflicts. In addition, Rhoades wanted to investigate whether the literature on children's reactions to interpersonal conflict is sufficiently large enough to warrant a systematic review and provide a theoretical background. The meta-analysis examined 17 articles and showed that cognition and negative affect were strongly related to child adjustment. Behavioural and physiological reactions to conflicts were also related, but not as strongly as cognition and negative affect. The author also found that the relationship between children's responses to interpersonal conflict and their internalizing behaviours was larger than with externalizing behaviours. Finally, there was no difference between genders, but a stronger association was found in older children. The conclusion of this particular study was essentially focusing on how important it is to the parental conflict, which is moderately related to the child adjustment. A limitation of this analysis is the small effect size, which should be considered as marital adjustment does not necessarily cause child behaviour problems. Instead they could have a bidirectional influence, that is, a child who exhibits problematic behaviour may in turn influence the parents' marital behaviour, which can then further impact the behaviour of the child. Additionally, there may be some other factors that influence the child's outcome when couples do not agree on the parenting styles.

One such variable could be the way in which the child is disciplined, especially in the presence of argumentative, hostile parents. Often, the child will imitate such behaviours and become defiant. Another way the child can cope with such a chaotic environment is one of withdrawing, not interacting and internalizing their problems. No matter what the environment may be, one of the important ways in which the child is directly affected is the way the parents confer discipline. Generally, in heterosexual couples, it is the mother who provides the majority of caregiving, as well as engaging in discipline. O'Leary and Vidair tested the hypothesis that the relationship between marital adjustment and children's behaviour problems is mediated by child-rearing disagreements. The results of the study showed that the children learned to be oppositional, defiant and aggressive when parents were showing externalizing behaviours, while alternatively, some children chose to be avoidant and withdrawn, mimicking the internalizing behaviours of their parents. The investigators' hypothesis was largely supported as mediating roles were found for child-rearing disagreements and overreactive discipline in child behaviour problems. In clinical practice, marital counsellors are often dealing with the impact of the couple's problems on their children. Therefore, the findings of the above study should be beneficial in illustrating the importance of instituting marital therapy in couples who are struggling with parental disagreements. Also, it is especially important that both parents are involved in such treatment, as marital harmony is an important aspect of parenting, both in the short and long term. This is especially applicable to those parents who are together and raising their children in a family environment.

Treatment Recommendations: How Do You Intervene?

Partner support is found to protect against not just perinatal mood disorders, but also depressive disorders in men. The prevention of psychiatric illness in one of the partners is dependent on the support he or she receives from the partner who is functioning well. Recently, two panels of experts in perinatal mental health, which consisted of 21 consumer advocates and 39 professionals, participated in a Delphi consensus study to establish how partners can support one another to reduce the risk of developing depression and anxiety specific to pregnancy and the postpartum period. In this study by Pilkington and colleagues, 214 recommendations were made with regard to how partners can support each other in reducing the risk of perinatal depression and anxiety. The results of this study showed that partner support was identified as a key protective factor against mood problems during pregnancy and after childbirth. They further went on to state that there were some specific techniques that would help couples interact with each other. These included developing acceptance, encouraging each other to take care of themselves and satisfaction with sexual relationships. Over and above the Delphi consensus study, there are some other techniques supported by empirical evidence such as positive communication, emotional closeness, emotional support and practical support in minimizing conflict. What was clear in this study was that partners appeared to prefer accessing support from each other and family, as opposed to resources outside the family. The authors concluded that the guidelines identified in their study could help new and expectant parents understand how to best support one another. In clinical practice, it is often seen that unless and until there is guidance provided to the couple, specifically with regard to how they should support one another, their interpersonal problems do not get resolved. We have a marital therapist at the Reproductive Mental Health Program who engages in one-to-one therapy, guiding couples through challenging times while the mother is going through perinatal depression. This can become an especially challenging issue to treat, i.e. the marital discord, if both partners suffer from psychiatric disorders. Moreover, in our programme, we also have group couples' therapy whereby the interactional patterns can be either validated or challenged in the presence of others who are going through similar difficulties. Years of clinical experience shows that the successful outcome of resolving marital differences is based on proper guidance and support which gives them a sense of hope for their future together.

Integrative behavioural couples therapy (IBCT) is a promising new treatment for couples' discord, according to Jacobsen and colleagues. They interviewed 21 couples who were experiencing marital distress and randomly assigned them to IBCT or traditional behavioural couples therapy (TBCT). In this sample, 80% of couples that received IBCT improved or recovered at the end of therapy compared to 64% of TBCT couples, thus concluding in this preliminary study that IBCT shows promise for couples that are experiencing discord. The IBCT model helps spouses accept challenging aspects of each other and uses unsolvable problems as vehicles to establish greater intimacy, whereas TBCT focuses on helping individuals change in accordance with their partners' complaints with active collaboration and compromise. A more recent literature review by Christiansen and

Doss backs the effectiveness of IBCT in Jacobson's earlier study. In addition, the review showed that IBCT resulted in better maintenance over 2 years post-treatment and that several real-life applications showed significant improvement. Therefore, this type of marital therapy shows promise as a therapeutic treatment for marital discord. Clearly, this type of therapy warrants further exploration, in the form of a randomized controlled trial.

Another method of treating marital distress is behavioural marital therapy. Behavioural marital therapy (BMT) is a technique that uses behavioural therapy and attempts to alleviate marital distress by increasing positive interactions between couples and decreasing the harmful interactions. A meta-analysis of 30 studies showed that those who received BMT had better outcomes compared to those who had no treatment, but that this treatment may have lower effect sizes than previously reported.

In conclusion, given the pervasive effects of relationship discord on the health of the partners as well as their children, it is imperative that health-care providers screen for and treat this issue in new parents. When untreated, relationship dysfunction can have intergenerationally detrimental effects on the family system. As such, the existence of dysfunctional dyadic relationships in new parents should not go unaddressed.

Take-Home Messages

1. Marital conflict can be intergenerationally transmitted, beginning with its roots in the family of origin. When unaddressed, inter-parental discord can have long-term consequences on children.
2. Sleep deprivation is a common in new parents and can increase disruptive partner relations, such as increased irritability, outburst of anger and blaming behaviours.
3. Marital discord and psychiatric disorders have been found to have a bidirectional longitudinal relationship.
4. Maternal employment status and paternal attitude towards child-rearing are connected to the level of satisfaction in a relationship.

5. In treating cognitive, behavioural, affective and physiological outcomes in new parents with psychiatric disorders, it is important to address relationship conflict.
6. Several effective psychological and behavioural treatments for relationships exist.

References

1. Amato PR, Cheadle JE. Parental divorce, marital conflict and children's behavior problems: a comparison of adopted and biological children. Soc Forces. 2008;86(3):1139–61.
2. American Psychiatric Association. Diagnostic and statistical manual of mental disorders (DSM-5®). USA: American Psychiatric Pub; 2013.
3. Cookston JT, Braver SL, Griffin WA, et al. Effects of the dads for life intervention on interparental conflict and coparenting in the two years after divorce. Fam Process. 2007;46(1):123–37.
4. Davies P, Windle M. Interparental discord and adolescent adjustment trajectories: the potentiating and protective role of intrapersonal attributes. Child Dev. 2001;72(4):1163–78.
5. Doss BD, Rhoades GK, Stanley SM. The effect of the transition to parenthood on relationship quality: an 8-year prospective study. J Pers Soc Psychol. 2009;96(3):601.
6. Faircloth WB, Cummings EM. Evaluating a parent education program for preventing the negative effects of marital conflict. J Appl Dev Psychol. 2008;29(2):141–56.
7. Helms-Erikson H. Marital quality ten years after the transition to parenthood: implications of the timing of parenthood and the division of housework. J Marriage Fam. 2001;63(4):1099–110.
8. Jacobson NS, Christensen A, Prince SE, et al. Integrative behavioral couple therapy: an acceptance-based, promising new treatment for couple discord. J Consult Clin Psychol. 2000;68(2):351.
9. Kluwer ES, Johnson MD. Conflict frequency and relationship quality across the transition to parenthood. J Marriage Fam. 2007;69(5):1089–106.
10. Krishnakumar A, Buehler C. Interparental conflict and parenting behaviors: a meta-analytic review. Fam Relat. 2000;49(1):25–44.
11. Lee CY, Doherty WJ. Marital satisfaction and father involvement during the transition to parenthood. Fathering. 2007;5(2):75.

12. Medina AM, Lederhos CL, Lillis TA. Sleep disruption and decline in marital satisfaction across the transition to parenthood. Fam Syst Health. 2009;27(2):153.
13. Meyer JM, Rutter M, Silberg JL, et al. Familial aggregation for conduct disorder symptomatology: the role of genes, marital discord and family adaptability. Psychol Med. 2000;30(4):759–74.
14. O'Leary SG, Vidair HB. Marital adjustment, child-rearing disagreements, and overreactive parenting: predicting child behavior problems. J Fam Psychol. 2005;19(2):208.
15. Perren S, Wyl A, Bürgin D, et al. Intergenerational transmission of marital quality across the transition to parenthood. Fam Process. 2005;44(4):441–59.
16. Pilkington P, Milne L, Cairns K, et al. Enhancing reciprocal partner support to prevent perinatal depression and anxiety: a Delphi consensus study. BMC Psychiatry. 2016;16(1):23.
17. Risdal D, Singer GH. Marital adjustment in parents of children with disabilities: a historical review and meta-analysis. Res Pract Persons Severe Disabl. 2004;29(2):95–103.
18. Schudlich TD, Cummings EM. Parental dysphoria and children's adjustment: marital conflict styles, children's emotional security, and parenting as mediators of risk. J Abnorm Child Psychol. 2007;35(4):627–39.
19. Shadish WR, Baldwin SA. Effects of behavioral marital therapy: a meta-analysis of randomized controlled trials. J Consult Clin Psychol. 2004;73(1):6–14.
20. Troxel WM, Matthews KA. What are the costs of marital conflict and dissolution to children's physical health? Clin Child Fam Psychol Rev. 2004;7(1):29–57.
21. Vance JC, Boyle FM, Najman JM, et al. Couple distress after sudden infant or perinatal death: a 30-month follow up. J Paediatr Child Health. 2002;38(4):368–72.
22. Whisman MA. Marital distress and DSM-IV psychiatric disorders in a population-based national survey. J Abnorm Psychol. 2007;116(3):638.
23. Whisman MA. Relationship discord and the prevalence, incidence, and treatment of psychopathology. J Soc Pers Relatsh. 2013;30(2):163–70.
24. Whisman MA, Uebelacker LA. Prospective associations between marital discord and depressive symptoms in middle-aged and older adults. Psychol Aging. 2009;24(1):184.

Chapter 7
Sexual Dysfunction in the New Father: Sexual Intimacy Issues

Dad's Story: Clinical Vignette

Joe and Elizabeth met while they were on a ski vacation. After a passionate romance of 6 months, Elizabeth got pregnant. She had a difficult first trimester with frequent spotting. This young couple, each 27 years of age, was advised by their physician not to engage in sexual intimacy for the next few weeks until Elizabeth was totally free of any spotting. Fearful of losing the baby, Elizabeth felt uncomfortable in continuing any sexual activity with Joe for the rest of the pregnancy. After the baby boy's birth, Elizabeth struggled with nursing issues for the first several months. Once breast-feeding was established properly, Joe and Elizabeth started to attempt sexual contact frequently. However, nursing the baby compromised sexual intimacy for Elizabeth. She could not transition easily from her maternal role to being a sexual partner. This was disappointing for Joe, who used to look forward to their sexual intimacy. Joe was unable to maintain an erection over a period of time, which significantly affected his self-esteem. Eventually, with any sexual contact, Joe found himself having very little or no desire for sexual contact with Elizabeth. He started to compete with the

(continued)

© Springer International Publishing AG 2018
S.K. Misri, *Paternal Postnatal Psychiatric Illnesses*,
https://doi.org/10.1007/978-3-319-68249-5_7

119

baby for her attention and affection. Over the next few months, Elizabeth became overly clingy towards the baby, and the constant bodily connection with the baby further isolated Joe from Elizabeth. He started to compete with the baby for her attention and affection. Attempts between the couple to be sexually intimate became increasingly difficult. Joe became short fused and controlling and sought out conflicts and arguments. Once in the middle of the night, Elizabeth found Joe intensely engrossed in front of a computer screen watching pornography. Confused and shocked, Elizabeth did not quite know how to handle this crisis. Afraid to rock the boat in what seemed to be a calm and stable marriage, she decided to continue to live in their family home and occupied the main part of the house, while Joe stayed in the basement. The couple sought counselling as they were both hopeful that they could salvage their relationship.

In therapy, it appeared that the love that Elizabeth and Joe had for each other was not an issue. They were both young, and they were attracted to one another in every other way. The only issue they were currently struggling with was some aspects of sexual dysfunction that bewildered them. They had not anticipated that the birth of the baby would change their sexual attraction for one another. It was unclear exactly what it was that was causing this difficulty, which was the focus of most of their therapy. A number of different ways of dealing with the pornographic addiction were also discussed. It appeared that the issue with looking online for sexual gratification was a recent development for Joe, who felt quite isolated and alone in their relationship during the pregnancy.

What was also difficult to comprehend for Joe during these sessions was that he was not particularly addicted to anything else in his life. He did not have an addictive personality, and he was quite well adjusted in most aspects of his life. However, his training as an IT specialist

(continued)

gave him a lot more freedom and access to what was available on the computer. Although he used this as an excuse to begin with, especially in his therapy sessions, what became clear is that it was his way of escaping from the reality of a temporarily non-existent sexual relationship. On the other hand, with Elizabeth, it appeared that she was no longer able to visualize her breasts as being sexual organs, but saw them only as a way of nurturing her child. She was having lots of difficulty with nursing in the beginning, which is why she was trying to protect the baby's feeding schedule by not engaging in sexual activity. For some reason, she related one activity to the other and thought that having sex would somehow compromise her ability to nurse her baby.

A number of different misconceptions about embarking on parenthood had led to the breakdown of sexual functioning for this young couple. It appeared that with proper therapy, eventually the sexual functioning became much better, especially in the area of erectile dysfunction, which was a significant issue for Joe. Eventually, the couple was able to engage in mutually satisfying sexual activity. They were glad that they sought help at the right time, in order to deal with what appeared to be a crisis situation for them.

DSM-5 Diagnosis

Male Hypoactive Sexual Desire Disorder

Criteria A: Persistently or recurrently deficient (or absent) sexual/erotic thoughts or fantasies and desires for sexual activity. The judgement of deficiency is made by the clinician taking into account factors that affect sexual functioning such as age and general and social-cultural context of the individual's life.

Criteria B: That the above symptoms have persisted for a minimum duration of approximately 6 months.

Criteria C: That these symptoms cause clinically significant distress in the individual.

Criteria D: Sexual dysfunction is not better explained by non-sexual mental disorder or as a consequence of severe relationship distress or other significant stressors and is not attributable to the effects of substance/medication or other medical conditions.

DSM-5 Criteria for Erection Disorder

Criteria A: At least one of the three following symptoms must be experienced on almost all or at least 75–100% of the occasions of sexual activity:

(i) *Marked difficulty in obtaining an erection during sexual activity*

(ii) *Marked difficulty in maintaining an erection until completion of sexual activity*

(iii) *Marked decrease in erectile rigidity*

Criteria B: Symptoms in Criteria A have persisted for approximately 6 months' duration.

Criteria C: Symptoms in Criteria A cause clinically significant distress in the individual.

Criteria D: Sexual dysfunction is not better explained by a non-sexual mental disorder or as a consequence of severe relationship distress or other significant stressors, i.e. substance/medication or other medical conditions.

Review of the Disorder

Introduction

It appears that there is not a lot in the literature addressing the issue of sexual difficulties that a couple might experience when a woman is pregnant and/or postpartum. In my clinical experience, in the first few months of the postpartum period and especially in the last trimester of pregnancy, it is not unusual for many couples to either decrease their sexual contact or at times abstain depending on circumstances during the pregnancy or in the postpartum period. On the other hand, it is not unusual for the occasional couple to increase sexual contact, especially in the last trimester of pregnancy. It appears in the case of Joe and Elizabeth that the total lack of sexual intimacy within a few months of knowing one another was one of the main factors that led to their eventual sexually dysfunctional relationship. However, there are many other factors to examine that affect sexuality during pregnancy and the postpartum period. In an article by Bitzer and Alder, the authors provided a biopsychosocial framework to understand the interaction between pregnancy, the postpartum period and sexuality. There are many important reasons why an understanding of the impact of pregnancy and postpartum on sexual functioning is needed. Many women do not feel safe having sex during pregnancy as they are afraid of hurting the baby. They are also worried about further complicating the pregnancy, and many experience a general decline in sexual activity. Other women also feel less attractive when they are pregnant, leading to less interest in sexual intercourse. A lot of women continue to be intimate in other ways, but intercourse is often practised less often, and this leads to less sexually content partners.

Transition to parenthood can be stressful and emotionally draining, a phase that serves a developmental function in the personalities of both parents, and includes healthy adjustments of sexual needs during pregnancy and also coping strategies. On a biological level, it appears that there are a lot of changes, both physical and psychological, with regard to general functioning. For instance, there is an increase in the levels of oestrogen and progesterone, as well as other hormones, which can impact sexual desire depending on the individual. There is also the impact of hormones on the connective tissue, pelvic structures and related flexibility, which can sometimes lead to less pleasurable sex. The psychological changes during pregnancy are also important to consider and address. For instance, there is a loss of independence once a woman becomes a mother. She can never go back to her pre-pregnancy level of functioning. She is now responsible for somebody else's life, therefore compromising her own autonomy. These conflictual feelings can cause a lot of anxiety, not necessarily pathological, but the wish to remain independent versus the joy of being a mother can often create emotional upheaval, both during pregnancy and after the birth of the baby. Studies in the past have also shown that marital satisfaction is likely to decrease after becoming parents. It can often be challenging to prepare for the triadic relationship between the couple and the new baby, while simultaneously continuing to maintain the successful dyadic relationship with a romantic partner. Some of these anxieties can appear during the last trimester of pregnancy as motherhood becomes imminent and there is no turning back. Sexual interest and coital activity often decline during the third trimester of pregnancy. Therefore, the complex interaction of biopsychosocial changes, both during pregnancy and postpartum, influences sexual interest and behaviours. Similarly, fathers go through a range of different degrees of sexual functioning throughout postpartum. For instance, many partners develop anxiety around initiating sexual contact with their partners who are on bed rest, or intermittently bleeding, or have other medical problems that accompany their pregnancy. It is not uncommon for a husband to watch childbirth and to make the transition from his wife being a mother into a sexual partner. However, many dads in therapy have expressed anxiety about having a sexual relationship with the mother of their newborn child. Additional complications of caesarean sections or significant vaginal tears can also lead to not having the desire to resume sexual intimacy.

In the last phases of pregnancy, for instance, anticipation and preparation for birth are often accompanied by marked emotional states, as fear of the unknown impacts a shift in mood. There are often feelings of ambivalence, emotional lability and a variety of other reactions that accompany the embarkation to motherhood. Often the body image of the mother changes because of the effects of pregnancy, over which she has no control.

In the postpartum period, the review by Bitzer and colleague found that in the first weeks postpartum, up to 3 months after the birth, 40% of women will still have little or no interest in sexual activity. Postpartum sexual problems are therefore relatively common. Individual responses to these changes can improve sexual life or can lead to sexual problems, dysfunction and difficulties. These problems can then have mid- to long-term negative impacts on the physical and mental health of women and their relationship/family development. The difference in sexual desire between partners is a critical factor. Therefore, sexual health care should be combined routinely with antenatal and postnatal care. The treating clinician should initiate the topic of sexual intimacy between partners so as to start a dialogue without feeling embarrassed or ashamed of the different feelings associated with sexual intimacy.

Epidemiology

The DSM-5 outlines the prevalence of male hyperactive sexual desire disorder, which varies depending on the country of origin, and the method of assessment. Approximately 6% of younger men between the ages of 18 and 24 and 41% of older men between the ages of 66 and 74 have problems with sexual desire; however, a persistent lack of interest in sex lasting for more than 6 months only affects a very small population of males, i.e. 1.8% between the ages of 16 and 44.

On the other hand, the prevalence of lifelong versus acquired erectile disorder remains unknown. There is a strong age-related increase, both in prevalence and incidence of problems of erection, particularly after age 50. Furthermore, DSM also outlines that anywhere between 13% and 21% of men between the ages of 40 and 80 complain of occasional problems with erection, whereas only 2% of men between the ages of 40 and 50 complain of frequent problems with erection. In an article by Beutel and colleagues, the authors aimed to review the epidemiology of sexual dysfunction in men which included lack of sexual desire, erectile dysfunction, disorders of ejaculation and orgasm and issues of sexual activity and satisfaction. Their findings were that sexual desire declines in men over 40 years of age, but sexual interest is maintained. They also found that erection problems were seen as bothersome by 77.6% of responders, but this perception decreased with age. Ejaculation problems were bothersome for over 50%; however men between the ages of 18 and 40 appeared to be more satisfied with their sexuality, compared to those over 60. Additionally, the presence of a partnership was an important factor with older men. The determinants of sexual dysfunction include urologic and andrologic as well as cardiovascular, metabolic, psychiatric and other comorbidities, which appear to be interrelated, especially when different health behaviours are examined. The authors concluded that there appears to be an interrelationship between risk factors for sexual dysfunction. They suggested that assessment should cover medical as well as psychological factors and also that interventions for sexual dysfunction should target multiple risk factors.

Risk Factors

Dr. Lori Brotto examined the applicability of the DSM-5 criteria for hypoactive sexual disorder in men by reviewing the prevalence and correlates, both qualitatively and quantitatively, on the experience of sexual desire.

She found that the prevalence of low desire ranged from 14% to 17% in older men and those who were likely to be in poorer health (e.g. due to alcohol or emotional problems), compared to 7% in those 18–29 years of age. Also, she found that there was comorbidity between depression and low sexual desire in men with infrequent sexual activity.

The association between low testosterone and hypoactive sexual disorder was significant in middle-aged men. Men with this particular disorder were also more likely to have depressed mood and hyperprolactinemia. They also had evidence of free-floating anxiety, some obsessive-compulsive traits and somatization. These individuals tended to have greater stress at work and more disturbed domestic relationships. Often, sex is used as a mood regulator, that is, depressed men feel validated if they make their partner happy because of a satisfactory sexual relationship. An interesting component of this article was the observation of difference of experiences in men versus women. For instance, men seek treatment at much older ages than women. However, both were likely to experience secondary sexual dysfunction, which in men usually accounted for erectile dysfunction and in women for subjective sexual arousal. Psychological factors included self-esteem and intimacy motivations.

The risk and prognostic factors described in DSM-5 for erectile dysfunction (ED) include alexithymia. In this condition, there are often deficits in cognitive functioning or processing of emotion. This is more common in men who are diagnosed with "psychogenic erectile dysfunction". Risk factors for acquired ED include smoking tobacco, lack of physical exercise, diabetes and age.

With regard to risk and prognostic factors for male hypoactive sexual disorder, DSM-5 describes temperamental, environmental, genetic and physiological factors which impact this specific type of sexual disorder. Mood and anxiety symptoms appear to be strong predictors of low desire in men. A man's self-image, his perception of his partner's sexual desire towards him, feelings of being emotionally connected and contextual variables may all negatively affect sexual desire.

Alcohol use increases the occurrence of low desire. Social and cultural contextual factors also should be considered. Finally, as far as the physiological and genetic aspects are concerned, endocrine disorders, such as hyperprolactinemia, are found to significantly affect sexual desire in men. It is unclear however whether this is due to these men having low levels of testosterone. In hypogonadal men, low desire is more common. Therefore, there may be a critical threshold below which testosterone will affect sexual desire in men.

Relationship Functioning and Sexual Desire

Interpersonal relationships go through different phases, depending on where the couple is in terms of their life circumstances. For instance, much more profound changes are expected when the couple becomes first-time parents. After the birth of the second or third child, the well-adjusted family may have fewer problems in this regard. The importance of interpersonal aspects of sexual desire disorders has been recognized since the earliest work on the topic of sexual dysfunction. Generally, marital distress, dissatisfaction or conflicts can cause or be an outcome of low sexual desire. The effects of marital satisfaction and power were examined by Brezsnyak and colleagues, in a population of husbands. They examined the association between marital satisfaction, marital power and sexual desire in a sample of 60 heterosexual community couples. They administered several specific questionnaires with regard to these issues. Their results showed that marital satisfaction predicted sexual desire both in husbands and wives and was not moderated by marital power. Secondly, the study also suggested that marital dissatisfaction may directly produce low sexual desire, resulting in withdrawal from the relationship. It is also possible that the existence of low sexual desire may cause a breakdown in the marital relationship. Higher congruence in the husband's desire and perceived balance of decision-making power correlated with higher sexual desire. Their conclusion was that marital dissatisfaction is associated with low sexual desire, whereas the opposite may not necessarily be true, i.e. that low sexual desire may not always cause marital problems. The limitation of this study included that the sexual dysfunction was not diagnosed in detail and that this was only applicable in heterosexual couples.

In another study by Corona, the researchers aimed to investigate primary reduced libido and secondary reduced libido. They studied 3714 men attending a clinic for the first time, between the ages of 53.2 ± 12 years. The results showed that the common dysfunctions seen in this population included reduced libido with comorbid ED, premature ejaculation and delayed ejaculation. Reduced libido by itself as an isolated condition was only present in approximately 5% of the sample. Secondary reduced libido was more universally as a result of hyperprolactinemia due to medical conditions, whereas primary reduced libido was more common in those with romantic relationship disturbances. Primary reduction here relates to those who do not have medical conditions, whereas secondary reduced libido is more applicable to those with issues such as hypogonadism and other medical conditions, as earlier suggested.

Marital Satisfaction

Conflicts within the family and couples can also determine male sexual functioning. In 2015, Boddi and colleagues studied men attending an outpatient clinic for sexual dysfunction. They aimed to evaluate the relationship between male sexual dysfunction (SD) and conflicts within the couple or family. About 3975 male patients were studied for conflicts within the family and couples using two standard questions: "Are there any conflicts at home?" and "Do you have a difficult relationship with your partner?" The results showed that family and couple conflicts were significantly associated with anxiety symptoms, depression as well as a higher risk of subjective and objective erectile dysfunction and hypoactive sexual desire. Family and partner conflict could potentially prolong or exacerbate sexual problems, irrespective of the original cause of the condition. Therefore, this study showed that conflicts within the family or within the direct relationship can be important contextual factors in the development of male sexual dysfunction. Another article by Moore and colleagues showed that late adulthood ED may be a result of medical complications, whereas early onset may be associated with psychosocial and relationship difficulties. In this particular study, 560 male patients from a sexual health clinic were studied to explore whether their erectile dysfunction was associated with psychosocial and adjustment problems.

There were three age categories that were examined: 18–39 years of age (early), 40–59 (middle) and over 60 (late). The researchers found that younger men reported less relationship satisfaction, greater depressive symptomatology and more negative reactions from female partners but also greater overall rating of their sex life, more frequent intercourse and better overall erectile functioning. The middle and late groups had significantly lower erectile functioning and less frequent intercourse than the early.

Pornography

Research suggests that the rapid rate of increase in sexual dysfunction, especially among men, is related to the surge in Internet pornography. Anxiety in general about sexual performance may compel people to rely on pornography as a sexual outlet. In 2014, Bronner and Ben-Zion reported that compulsive Internet pornography users whose tastes had escalated to extreme hard-core pornography sought help for low sexual desire during partnered sex. A literature review done by Park and colleagues in 2016, which investigated factors behind the recent increase in sexual dysfunction, showed that pornography is suggested to be a "supernormal stimulus", that is, an exacerbated imitation of what we are evolutionarily wired to pursue in terms of constant novelty, availability and variability. Pornography could be a self-reinforcing activity and can also increase the incentive salience, which refers to hyperactivity to Internet cues and hypoactivity to partnered sex. It often can result in sexual conditioning, which does not necessarily transfer to real-life sexual activity, therefore leading to a decrease in sexual functioning overall. Terminating Internet pornography use is sometimes sufficient to reverse negative effects. This review concluded that the increased availability and use of pornography may be important relevant factors which impact the prevalence of sexual dysfunction.

With regard to the significance of heavy pornography involvement and how it impacts the romantic partner, a study by Bergner and Bridges showed that the discovery of heavy pornography use by a partner appears to create feelings of undesirability and distress in some women. In their study, Bergner and Bridges aimed to investigate the effects of the discovery, significance and experience of women with partners who are heavy pornography users. One hundred personal letters posted on Internet messengers by spouses, fiancées and girlfriends of men perceived to be involved in heavy pornography use were studied. They found that the discovery of pornography use was a traumatic event that changed the women's view of the relationship, themselves and their partners. These women also felt betrayed, sexually undesired, isolated and/or unloved. Often these women felt that they were not understood and that they had been lied to or that they had themselves been living a lie or viewing their partners as being liars. Often, the partners were seen as unloving, selfish or inadequate husbands.

For Elizabeth, it was important to understand that although she felt that she was being betrayed by her husband, he was not really addicted to pornography and it was a temporary way of escaping from the reality of non-intimacy in their relationship. This was a very important factor in making this relationship work, as often in couples where a partner uses pornography in an addictive manner, they are either perceived as being sick or bad. It appears that this sort of dichotomy is often related to relationship outcome. Another important factor is whether the husband is repentant and apologetic about using this modality of escape. It appears that with Joe, once he understood the implications of where this type of behaviour could lead, the change in his thinking towards sexual intimacy was helpful in stopping any further viewing of Internet pornography.

Our knowledge to date on the sharp rise in sexual dysfunction and low sexual desire in men under 40 and its relationship to Internet pornography is an important area to research and then offer intervention. One method of treating these individuals is the use of acceptance and commitment therapy (ACT). The efficacy of this type of treatment was evaluated by researchers who treated problematic pornography with ACT. This is a small set of case reports consisting of six adult males who reported how pornography use impacted their quality of life. They were treated with eight 1.5-h sessions of ACT. Five out of the six patients had clinically notable reductions in pornography viewing after treatment, with the sixth showing some reduction. At 3 months, most of them continued to show reduction, with one who went back to pretreatment level. Quality of life increased by 8% after treatment, and after 3 months, by 16%. The conclusion of this study was that the acceptance and commitment therapy appears to be a well-tolerated treatment for problematic pornography viewing.

Another recent and interesting study involved a case series of men treated with paroxetine in combination with cognitive behaviour therapy (or CBT) for treatment of problematic pornography use. This was a 2- to 4-week trial which resulted in decreased libido after treatment as well as delayed ejaculation. Within 10 weeks, these individuals reported libido close to normal, with decreased levels of anxiety and decreased use of pornography. After 12–14 weeks, however, new sexual behaviours emerged, including paid sexual relations, and one had an extra-marital affair. Therefore, the authors concluded that paroxetine may have some short-term reduction of problematic pornographic use, but new behaviours may emerge, and that further investigation in this area was necessary before any conclusions could be drawn on a general basis.

Treatment Recommendations: How Do You Intervene?

A variety of collaborative approaches are recommended when it comes to treating sexual dysfunction. These interventions should include participation by nurses, physicians, sexual health educators (where available) and finally also the sexual partner. The management and improvement in overall quality of sex life and the variety of related therapies are evolving. Assisting with timely treatment and rehabilitation of sex life in order to help couples achieve a better quality of life is the goal in treating sexual dysfunction, both in males and females. It is important to identify the risk factors that contribute to the development of this troubling reality for many couples and to address any unhealthy lifestyle, medical, drug or substance use and/or psychological issues and to not forget the impact of marital functioning. The concept of treating the couple together is now a commonly accepted practice, especially in sexual medicine clinics.

The role of the sexual partner in managing erectile dysfunction was outlined by Li and colleagues in 2016 in a review article which explored this specific association. They also looked at the management and improvement of sex life quality. The key points of this review were that the affected men often avoided talking about their problem or were unwilling to accept it and that the sex life quality was often affected. This could include the frequency of female orgasm, which correlated with severity of ED and/or lack of intimacy. Satisfaction of the sexual partner also decreased as the partners often felt rejected or suspicious.

This article also highlighted the fact that physicians often feel uncomfortable when conducting sexual history interviews especially with women and vice versa. Reduced communication and acquisition of sexual history was found to be an important factor in the maintenance of sexual dysfunction. Understanding of ED was highly important in encouraging the proper treatment and support of the couple. Another interesting observation in this study was couples whose ED medications were less time dependent felt more satisfied in general. The conclusion of the study was that the sexual partners of men with ED played an important role in the management and improvement of sex life quality. Secondly, the concept of treating the couple as a unit is a common practice and an important one to achieve optimal outcomes of treatment.

The presently available treatments for sexual dysfunction often lack proper methodological interventions, which can affect the accuracy of the effectiveness of any given treatment.

Frequently there is also a lack of clarification of the differential diagnosis for sexual dysfunction. Therefore, the outcome of the treatment does not have a clearly specified target, which makes evaluation difficult. One of the first studies that used cognitive behaviour therapy was to evaluate the sexual response of low subjective arousal in women. Based on the results of this study, its applicability to male sexual dysfunction was undertaken, although, at this point, these studies are still sparse. The loss of sexual desire has been considered to be one of the most difficult sexual dysfunctions to treat in both men and women. The efficacy of psychological intervention for sexual dysfunction was reviewed recently through meta-analysis of available studies from 1980 to 2009. A total of 28 randomized controlled studies comparing psychological intervention with a wait list were included in this analysis. The psychological interventions were shown to especially improve symptom severity for women with hypoactive sexual desire disorder and orgasmic disorder. However, no clear evidence from randomized controlled trials was found for other sexual dysfunctions, namely, erectile dysfunction, premature ejaculation, vaginismus and mixed sexual dysfunction. This meta-analysis also showed that male hypoactive sexual disorder was not well studied. Clearly, more studies are needed for males with regard to this type of cognitive behavioural intervention. While the meta-analysis focused on randomized controlled trials, in clinical practice, the use of techniques such as education, focusing on partner dynamics and subjective feelings associated with genital response are some of the simple techniques that are usually helpful in guiding the couple through their sexual difficulties.

In a study done in 2001 by McCabe, a cognitive behaviour programme for sexual dysfunction was evaluated. The study included 45 males and 54 females. The most common disorder in males was found to be ED, while in females it was lack of sexual interest. Therapy was found to be successful in 53.3% of males and was most likely to be effective in those with premature ejaculation. They were found to have a more positive attitude towards sex, which appeared to be more enjoyable, and participants were less likely to feel as though they were sexual failures. This study also demonstrated that both males and females who need intervention for sexual dysfunction may have a variety of problems. If the problems are long-standing, then they are generally not easily treatable, and short-term cognitive behaviour therapy is not effective if the arousal and desire phase has been an issue for a long time. The study showed that it is important to develop more intensive pro-grammes for change in lifestyle, cognitions and relationships of patients with overall sexual dysfunction. Often combining psychotherapy and pharmacotherapy is effective. Especially given the availability of medications for ED disorder in males, the combination of pharmacotherapy and psychotherapy appears to be superior to any of the interventions on their own.

With regard to pharmacological treatment, phosphodies-terase 5 inhibitors (PDE5Is) are one class of medicine which appears to be effective in the treatment of ED. As earlier stated, this is one of the sexual dysfunctions that is most com-monly prevalent in men between the ages of 40 and 70 and is reportedly experienced by up to about 50% of men. Therefore, it has substantive influence on the quality of a person's life. PDE5Is are the first-line medication treatments for ED. Presently, seven different types of PDE5Is are available in a variety of dosages and formulations. Chen and colleagues recently conducted a systematic review and meta-analysis, which included 82 trials, totalling more than 47,000 patients, to study the efficacy of PDE5I and also adverse event analy-sis. The results showed that sildenafil 50 mg (Viagra) had the greatest efficacy but also the highest rate of overall adverse events. Tadalafil 10 mg (Cialis) had intermediate efficacy but had the lowest overall rate of adverse events. The other most common medications are vardenafil and avanafil 100 mg, which had similar overall adverse events but markedly lower efficacy. Finally, udenafil 100 mg had similar efficacy to tadalafil 10 mg but higher adverse event rates. The conclusion of this study was that for those with prioritizing efficacy, Viagra was the treatment of choice. With regard to tolerabil-ity, Cialis was the first choice with udenafil in the second place. This important meta-analysis essentially shows that the clinicians will have to choose medications on a case-by-case basis. While some medications are highly effective, the related adverse events can be an issue, while for others, the effectiveness may not be as great, but the tolerability profile is better. Cost also appears to be an important consideration when these treatments are recommended. Therefore, a variety of therapeutic treatment options should be explored.

Take-Home Messages

1. Denial of sexual dysfunction is a common phenomenon.
2. Conflicts within the family or within the direct relationship can be important contextual factors in the development of male sexual dysfunction.
3. Research suggests the increased rate of sexual dysfunction, especially among men, is related to the surge in the usage of Internet pornography.
4. Physicians are often uncomfortable in eliciting sexual functioning in their overall assessments of patients, both male and female.
5. Sexual dysfunction is a shared health-care problem where physicians, nurses and educators need to share responsibility.
6. New treatment approaches include sexual/psychoeducation, phosphodiesterase 5 inhibitors (PDE5Is), cognitive behaviour therapy and couples' therapy.
7. It is also important to pay attention to comorbid medical and psychiatric disorders and treat them.

References

1. American Psychiatric Association. Diagnostic and statistical manual of mental disorders (DSM-5®). USA: American Psychiatric Pub; 2013.
2. Bergner RM, Bridges AJ. The significance of heavy pornography involvement for romantic partners: research and clinical implications. Sex Marital Ther. 2002;28(3):193–206.

3. Beutel ME, Weidner W, Brähler E. Epidemiology of sexual dysfunction in the male population. Andrologia. 2006;38(4):115–21.
4. Bogren LY. Changes in sexuality in women and men during pregnancy. Arch Sex Behav. 1991;20(1):35–45.
5. Brezsnyak M, Whisman MA. Sexual desire and relationship functioning: the effects of marital satisfaction and power. J Sex Marital Ther. 2004;30(3):199–217.
6. Brotto LA. The DSM diagnostic criteria for hypoactive sexual desire disorder in men. J Sex Med. 2010;7(6):2015–30.
7. DiBartolo PM, Barlow DH. Perfectionism, marital satisfaction, and contributing factors to sexual dysfunction in men with erectile disorder and their spouses. Arch Sex Behav. 1996;25(6):581–8.
8. Fedele D, Bortolotti A, Coscelli C, et al. Erectile dysfunction in type 1 and type 2 diabetics in Italy. Int J Epidemiol. 2000;29(3):524–31.
9. Gola M, Potenza MN. Paroxetine treatment of problematic pornography use: a case series. J Behav Addict. 2016;5(3):529–32.
10. Goldstein I, Young JM, Fischer J, et al. Vardenafil, a new phosphodiesterase type 5 inhibitor, in the treatment of erectile dysfunction in men with diabetes. Diabetes Care. 2003;26(3):777–83.
11. Gresser U, Gleiter CH. Erectile dysfunction: comparison of efficacy and side effects of the PDE-5 inhibitors sildenafil, vardenafil and tadalafil-review of the literature. Eur J Med Res. 2002;7(10):435–46.
12. Landripet I, Štulhofer A. Is pornography use associated with sexual difficulties and dysfunctions among younger heterosexual men? J Sex Med. 2015;12(5):1136–9.
13. Li H, Gao T, Wang R. The role of the sexual partner in managing erectile dysfunction. Nat Rev Urol. 2016;13(3):168–77.
14. McCabe MP. Evaluation of a cognitive behavior therapy program for people with sexual dysfunction. Sex Marital Ther. 2001;27(3):259–71.
15. Moore TM, Strauss JL, Herman S, et al. Erectile dysfunction in early, middle, and late adulthood: symptom patterns and psychosocial correlates. Sex Marital Ther. 2003;29(5):381–99.
16. Müller MJ, Ruof J, Graf-Morgenstern M, et al. Quality of partnership in patients with erectile dysfunction after sildenafil treatment. Pharmacopsychiatry. 2001;34(3):91–5.
17. Nelson CJ. The impact of male sexual dysfunction on the female partner. Curr Sex Health Rep. 2006;3(1):37–41.
18. Nicolosi A, Moreira ED, Shirai M, et al. Epidemiology of erectile dysfunction in four countries: cross-national study of

the prevalence and correlates of erectile dysfunction. J Urol. 2003;61(1):201–6.

19. Park BY, Wilson G, Berger J, et al. Is Internet pornography causing sexual dysfunctions? A review with clinical reports. Behav Sci. 2016;6(3):17.

20. Rust J, Golombok S, Collier J. Marital problems and sexual dysfunction: how are they related? Br J Psychiatry. 1988;152(5):629–31.

21. Schiavi RC, White D, Mandeli J, et al. Effect of testosterone administration on sexual behavior and mood in men with erectile dysfunction. Arch Sex Behav. 1997;26(3):231–41.

22. Schmidt HM, Munder T, Gerger H, et al. Combination of psychological intervention and phosphodiesterase-5 inhibitors for erectile dysfunction: a narrative review and meta-analysis. J Sex Med. 2014;11(6):1376–91.

23. Seftel AD, Sun P, Swindle R. The prevalence of hypertension, hyperlipidemia, diabetes mellitus and depression in men with erectile dysfunction. J Urol. 2004;171(6):2341–5.

24. Simons JS, Carey MP. Prevalence of sexual dysfunctions: results from a decade of research. Arch Sex Behav. 2001;30(2):177–219.

25. Siu SC, Lo SK, Wong KW, et al. Prevalence of and risk factors for erectile dysfunction in Hong Kong diabetic patients. Diabet Med. 2001;18(9):732–8.

26. Stack S, Wasserman I, Kern R. Adult social bonds and use of internet pornography. Soc Sci Q. 2004;85(1):75–88.

27. Twohig MP, Crosby JM. Acceptance and commitment therapy as a treatment for problematic internet pornography viewing. Behav Ther. 2010;41(3):285–95.

Chapter 8
Paternal Substance Use: Finding Solace in Drugs and Alcohol

Dad's Story: Clinical Vignette

Adam was a 35-year-old stock broker from New York who met Daniella while holidaying in Canada. They fell in love right away and decided to get married within a short time of meeting one another. Daniella, an artist who loved poetry and nature, was a dreamer of sorts; she loved the outdoors, the ocean and the mountains. They both loved to ski and kayak. An unexpected pregnancy changed the couple's lifestyle of exploring and enjoying nature. Earlier in her pregnancy, Daniella was able to join Adam on different hikes and camp enthusiastically. However, in the second trimester, on and off cramps led to more physical restrictions. At some point, Adam began going out alone and enjoying his life outside of their new, cosy apartment. Daniella gave birth to a premature baby at 30 weeks. Adam's immediate response was one of fear and apprehension. He felt lost and confused as his life changed dramatically from being a single, carefree, inde-pendent man to that of a father of a newborn in the intensive care unit. Daniella and baby Zoe spent the first few weeks after the birth at the hospital. Meanwhile,

(continued)

© Springer International Publishing AG 2018
S.K. Misri, *Paternal Postnatal Psychiatric Illnesses*,
https://doi.org/10.1007/978-3-319-68249-5_8

Adam became increasingly despondent and aloof. He slowly stopped involving himself in the welfare of both his baby and his wife. Daniella hoped that this behaviour would change once their baby was discharged home.

Unfortunately, Adam's absences from home increased. Based on his escalating erratic behaviours and attitude, Daniella began to suspect that Adam was abusing drugs of some sort but had no proof. Gradually, Adam started staying out late at night and appearing at home around 4 or 5 in the morning. Later on, it became commonplace for Adam to stay out for two or three nights in a row. One day, in desperation, Daniella called her mother-in-law in New York, who informed Daniella that her son had been in treatment for drugs and alcohol abuse as a teenager but to her knowledge had overcome his addiction issues. Daniella recalled that earlier in their relationship, Adam had casually mentioned that he smoked marijuana and used cocaine recreationally during his early adulthood. With the passage of time, Adam became increasingly edgy and inaccessible and eventually left for New York without prior notice and without talking to Daniella. The demands of being a father of a premature infant resulted in a relapse of Adam's substance abuse. Escape was his only way of coping with his mental turmoil.

Throughout her marriage to Adam, Daniella was aware of his "up and down moods". At times, he was happy, gregarious and outgoing, while at other times she found him sulking, distressed and uncommunicative. Especially in the first few months of their relationship, she found these mood changes to be actually quite exciting, as there was a part of Adam that was unpredictable and mysterious. She assumed the mood shifts to be part of his personality and his way of coping with life in general. However, with advancing pregnancy, these mood fluctuations escalated to different levels, marked by irritability and prickliness. Other than a couple of male friends who he hung out with most of the time, Adam was

(continued)

quite socially withdrawn and was also frequently restless, especially in the third trimester of her pregnancy; he began to isolate himself and became emotionally unavailable over time.

One night, when Adam came home around midnight, Daniella saw him stumble on the floor drenched in perspiration. He was showing a great deal of distress with intense anxiety and high pulse rate. Afraid, and not knowing how she should deal with the ongoing state of affairs, Daniella decided to phone his mother and express concerns about her son's now unpredictable conduct and unknown activities. The next morning when Adam got up, he was very suspicious. He started to pick on Daniella about issues that were completely inconsequential in an aggressive manner; he became argumentative and was almost convinced that there was some sort of conspiracy against him. Confused and upset, Daniella did not understand what was going on and how to respond to this volatile outburst and paranoia. When such episodes began to reoccur more frequently, Daniella began to worry about her safety as well as that of Zoe. The final straw that propelled her to take more decisive action was when Adam arrived one morning after an absence of 2 days, agitated and almost noncoherent. He was restless and on edge; he complained of unpleasant dreams, exhaustion and extraordinary fatigue. At this point, he was also exhibiting impaired judgement in general and was stating that his life did not make sense; she knew at once that this was a crisis situation which needed urgent intervention. Daniella took Adam to the walk-in clinic, and the physician there confirmed that Adam was going through cocaine withdrawal.

Adam's earlier developmental history was traumatic and troubled. It appears that his father was not present in his life to any notable degree. Daniella learned from Adam's mother that drug addiction and alcoholism ran in Adam's family and that his father was often very drunk and aggressive. This was witnessed by Adam when he was

(continued)

growing up. Additionally, Adam witnessed verbal abuse between his parents. The mother and father split up when Adam was 6 years old; his mother raised him almost entirely alone. Adam was spoilt and indulged terribly. He learned to cope with stresses in his life by excessive drinking as a teenager; in his college years, he went on to smoke marijuana, and finally, when he became a financial success, cocaine abuse began. Adam's mother made repeated attempts to get him help in New York, but they were met with denial, resistance and non-compliance. Eventually, after an inpatient admission to an addiction facility, Adam became clean prior to meeting Daniella. He concentrated on his business and travelled extensively; he did well for himself by keeping away from drug and alcohol use and maintaining mental stability.

His way of escaping his own early childhood struggles was now playing out in his adult life and his new identity as a father, as he had not dealt with his conflict-laden relationship with his own father. Now, being a new father of a baby to whom he could not relate, he felt hopeless and helpless. Adam resorted to his familiar ways of coping with stress, which were maladaptive. The demands of being a father of a premature infant resulted in a relapse of Adam's substance abuse. Escape was his only way of coping with his mental turmoil.

DSM-5 Diagnosis

Diagnostic Criteria: Stimulant Use Disorder

A. A pattern of amphetamine-type substance, cocaine or other similar use leading to clinically significant impairment or distress as manifested by at least two of the following occurring within a 12-month period:

   1. The stimulant is often taken in large amounts or over a longer period than was intended.

2. There is a persistent desire or unsuccessful effort to cut down or control stimulant use.

3. A great deal of time is spent in activities necessary to obtain the stimulant, use the stimulant or recover from its effects.

4. Craving or a strong desire or urge to use the stimulant.

5. Recurrent stimulant use resulting in a failure to fulfil major role or obligation at work, in school or at home.

6. Continued stimulant use, despite having persistent or recurrent social or interpersonal problems caused by the effects of the stimulant.

7. Important social, occupational or recreational activities are given up or reduced because of the stimulant use.

8. Recurrent stimulant use in situations in which it is physically hazardous.

9. Stimulant use is continued despite knowledge of having persistent or recurrent physical or psychological problems likely to have been caused or exacerbated by the stimulant.

10. Tolerance as defined by either of the following:

    (a) A need for markedly increased amounts of the stimulant to achieve intoxication or desired effect

    (b) A markedly diminished effect with continued use of the same amount of stimulant

11. Withdrawal as manifested by either of the following:

    (a) Characteristic withdrawal syndrome for the stimulant.

    (b) The stimulant is taken to relieve or avoid withdrawal symptoms.

Review of the Disorder

Introduction

Research shows that alcohol use runs in families, with 40–60% of risk variants explained by genetic influences. Moreover, a three- to fourfold increase in risk has been observed in children of individuals with alcohol use disorder, even when these children were given up for adoption at birth and raised by adoptive parents who did not have the disorder. Often there appears to be simultaneous comorbid abuse of several substances. That is, those who are found to abuse stimulants often also drink alcohol excessively and/or have a high vulnerability associated with use of other substances.

Epidemiology

As per the DSM-5, in the United States, the 12-month prevalence rate of alcohol use disorder is estimated to be 4.6% among 12- to 17-year-olds and 8.5% among adults aged 18 years and older. Rates of the disorder are greater among adult men, rising to about 12.4%, compared to adult women where the prevalence rate is considerably lower at 4.9%. With increasing age, i.e. individuals 65 years of age and older, it appears that the alcohol abuse rates drop to around 1.5%.

With regard to prevalence rates of cocaine use, the estimated 12-month prevalence in the United States is about 0.2% among 12- to 17-year-olds and 0.3% among individuals aged 18 years and older. It also happens to be lowest in those between the ages of 45 and 64, at around 0.1%. It also appears that the prevalence of cocaine use is greater in the Native American population compared to the African-American, Hispanic, White and Asian-American populations, specifically in the age group of 8- and 9-year-olds.

A study by Merline examined substance use among adults 35 years of age. They aimed to determine the prevalence of substance use at the beginning of midlife by using data from the "Monitoring the Future" Study. In this study, individuals were followed on a regular basis once every 2 years, until the age of 35. These individuals had abused cigarettes or alcohol, marijuana, cocaine and/or prescription drugs. The results of the study showed that 26% of the men smoked, 32% were involved in heavy drinking, 13% abused marijuana, 6% abused cocaine and 7% abused prescription drugs. The study also showed that men had higher rates of drinking, marijuana and cocaine use, and those with college degrees were less likely to use illicit substances. If participants had tried any illicit drugs other than marijuana by their senior year of high school, they were five times more likely to misuse cocaine at age 35. These study findings suggest that for most people, the foundation for later substance use is set up by the time they finish grade school. This was no different for Adam who was partying during his teenage years, gradually progressing to marijuana and then cocaine by the time he reached adulthood.

It is not unusual to find co-occurrence of substance use disorders and mood and anxiety disorders, which was also noticeable throughout Daniella's relationship with Adam. The National Epidemiologic Survey on Alcohol and Related Conditions was recently conducted, using DSM-4 definitions. The aim of this study was to investigate the comorbidity between substance use disorders and mood and anxiety issues. Interestingly enough, the study results showed that the 12-month prevalence rates of substance use disorder, alcohol use and drug use were 9.35%, 8.46% and, 2%, respectively. The 12-month association of substance use disorder and mood and anxiety disorders was 84.8%. Among the anxiety disorders, the results showed that panic disorder with agoraphobia was most strongly related to substance abuse.

In conclusion, the study highlighted the comorbidity between mood/anxiety disorders and substance use disorders. It appears to be a bidirectional relationship in that those who have a psychiatric problem of depression and anxiety are more susceptible to using substances; but on the other hand, those with primary diagnoses of substance use can also have concurrent psychiatric problems such as depression and/or anxiety. Therefore, it is important that clinicians who are involved in treating these individuals address substance abuse and psychiatric disorders at the same time. It is not uncommon for clinicians to first stabilize the substance use disorder before an attempt is made to treat mood and anxiety disorders. Often, this is required in order to increase the therapeutic alliance and also adherence to treatment recommendations.

Comorbidities

Comorbidity of substance use with other psychiatric conditions is frequently encountered in clinical practice. The concurrent use of more than one substance is also commonly seen in populations that seek help. Comorbid substance use may stem from genetic and psychosocial factors, which have been well documented in several studies. Major depressive episodes, generalized anxiety disorder and antisocial personality disorder often occur comorbidly with substance use disorders such as marijuana or alcohol.

Gender plays an important role in how these comorbidities occur and also with regard to those who seek treatment versus those who do not. For instance, females will have more comorbidity with certain psychiatric conditions than their male counterparts. This includes generalized anxiety disorder as well as major depressive episodes (MDE). Lian Yu Chen and colleagues in 2016 compared the substance use (SUD) treatment patterns and barriers to treatment among men and women with and without comorbidity with major depressive episodes. Data from 227,123 adult participants in the National Survey of Drug Use and Health from 2005 to 2010 was collected. Both men and women with comorbid MDE were more likely to use SUD services compared to those without MDE. Gender also seems to have modified the treatment patterns. For instance, males with SUD/MDE had a higher likelihood of emergency room visits and the use of inpatient services than females. The results also showed that the barriers to substance use treatments were remarkably similar for males and females, both for SUD with or without MDE. The conclusion of the study was that comorbidity with MDE appeared to be an important predictor of service utilization and perceived need for SUD treatment, both in men and women. The finding that the types of treatments needed for men and women varied has significant implications for the design of gender-specific SUD treatment programmes. One explanation for this finding, suggested by the authors, was that there was a greater severity of SUD when it was associated with comorbid psychiatric disorders. It is also possible that the use of mental health services, due to a depressive episode, may lead to accessing information about SUD in these individuals and thereby enabling direct treatment referral for these patients. The other possibility is that those who have comorbid MDE and substance use disorder issues are more aware of their changing moods than those who do not have the condition of MDE.

With regard to gender differences in this particular study, it appears that the male participants were more likely than females to be hospitalized. This may have to do with the medical conditions that may comorbidly occur in individuals who have long-standing chronic struggles with SUD. Another interesting point raised in this study is the attitudinal barriers to treatment sought by individuals. It appears that a lot of participants did not want to use professional help due to pessimistic treatment attitudes, as well as financial barriers. This particular issue seems to be crucial for both those who suffer from SUD with or without MDE. Therefore, it is important to instil hope in these individuals who are in and out of hospitals on a regular basis, especially in facilities where there is proximity to low-income demographics that are abusing substances in a chronic manner.

In another study by Brook et al., the researchers examined longitudinal associations between comorbid cigarette, alcohol and marijuana use and other psychopathologies such as antisocial personality disorder, major depressive episodes or generalized anxiety disorder in adulthood. Their participants were a random, community-based sample from the Children and Adults in the Community Study. Data were collected at six different time points from 1983 to 2006 from 607 adults. The researchers found that the participants could be grouped into five different categories: (1) those with HHH (these were individuals who were chronically using cigarettes, alcohol and marijuana), (2) DDD (those with delayed/late-starting cigarette, alcohol and marijuana use), (3) LML (those with low cigarette use or non-smokers, moderate alcohol use and occasional marijuana use), (4) HMN (chronic smoking, moderate alcohol use, but no marijuana use) and (5) NON (occasional alcohol use only). They compared those in the NON group, those who occasionally used alcohol only, to those who were chronically using alcohol, marijuana and cigarettes, the HHH group. They found that the NON group had significantly greater odds for never having depression, anxiety and/or anti-social personality disorder. Those in the DDD, LML and HMN groups had weaker or less consistent associations with the three psychiatric comorbidities, as compared to the HHH group. The researchers concluded that the long-term concur-rent use of more than one substance was associated with both externalizing and internalizing psychiatric disorders in adults. This is an important finding with regard to how Adam's sub-stance use issues played out as an adult. It is quite possible that after he witnessed the violence in his home, he had a gradual onset of fluctuating mood symptoms that were never diagnosed. It is also probable that he was anxious as a child, being affected by the uncertainty within his household that led to tension and stress over a number of years. A lot of indi-viduals, especially males, do not go for help for psychological symptoms on their own. Generally, it would be the use of substances that would lead them to seek help in the emer-gency room, as was the case with Adam. This study validates the struggles that Adam went through trying to deal with his SUD over a number of years.

The comorbidity between attention deficit hyperactivity disorder (ADHD) and substance use disorders is an interest-ing one. It is well known that ADHD occurs comorbidly with SUD much higher frequency than many other psychiatric disorders. Therefore, substance use disorders in these indi-viduals are not unusual. Studies also show that ADHD and SUD independently enhance the risk of comorbidity with mood and anxiety disorders, as well as personality disorders. Therefore, it is important for health-care providers to focus on various aspects of substance use disorder, including those with specific symptoms of ADHD. In an attempt to study this association, a study done by van Emmerik-van Oortmerssen and colleagues determined the comorbidity patterns in treat-ment-seeking substance use disorders with or without ADHD.

They obtained data from a cross-sectional international ADHD and substance use prevalence study with 1205 treatment-seeking SUD patients from 47 treatment centres in ten countries. They used structural diagnostic assessments to diagnose the disorders. The study findings showed that the prevalence of adult ADHD in the SUD sample was 13.9 and that antisocial personality disorder, bipolar disorder, major depressive disorder and current hypomanic episodes in patients with alcohol as the primary substance of use were all more prevalent in participants with threshold ADHD compared to subthreshold ADHD. Additionally, the study found that 75% of adult SUD patients with ADHD had a minimum of one other comorbid disorder compared to only 37% of SUD patients without ADHD. The conclusion of this study was that treatment-seeking SUD patients with ADHD were at a higher risk for additional externalizing disorders such as bipolar disorder, major depressive disorder and personality disorders. It could be that this is due to shared vulnerability for this type of psychopathology and this finding again strongly emphasizes the need for further integration of addiction treatment with general mental health services.

In summary, it appears that with new fathers who present with substance use disorders, whether in a crisis situation and/or with other comorbid conditions such as anxiety or depression, the clinician needs to be attentive to the possibility of comorbidity between these conditions. Often, there is a longitudinal history of psychiatric conditions that go unattended, which may resurface in the form of substance use disorders. On the other hand, over a number of years, patients with chronic substance use disorders also develop other comorbidities which do not get treated. The message here is that the comorbidity between several of these psychiatric conditions and SUD is more the norm than not. In the case of Adam, eventually after he was discharged from the treatment programme, a lot of his mood and anxiety issues were addressed, especially those that related to becoming a new father and within the context of a relatively new relationship.

Risk Factors

Presently, our knowledge with regard to the risk factors associated with substance use in young adults is sparse. However, a few available studies show that there are some specific risk factors that seem to be associated with increased substance use. A study of risk and protective factors of substance use in emerging adulthood done by Stone and colleagues in 2012 showed that males were more likely than females to abuse substances and that low socioeconomic status as a child increases the risk. The study also showed that children of alcoholics were more likely to be at risk. However, personality characteristics may be a mediating factor. Those who exhibit sensation-seeking behaviours, low levels of planning, impulsive behaviours or coping techniques or neurobehavioural inhibition are more likely to be at risk. With regard to other risk factors, history of abuse and neglect, especially paternal neglect in alcoholics, appears to be an important risk factor. This appears to be the case with Adam's developmental history, as he was almost abandoned by his biological father, in addition to his genetic vulnerability to substance abuse. This study also showed that fathers generally did not change their substance use habits after the birth of a child, whereas mothers did. This is an important point to consider, as the father's continued abuse of substances over a period of time can have short- and long-term impacts on the developing child. For instance, a longitudinal register-based study on mental disorders and harmful substance use was well documented in a Finnish national register. The researchers measured psychiatric disorders at 7–12 years and psychiatric disorders and substance use at 13–17 years of age. In this study, they found that the parental substance use was significantly associated with mental health issues and substance disorder in adolescents but not in young children. Furthermore, in this study maternal substance use was found to have a larger effect on the offspring than the fathers. The researchers concluded that because maternal substance use had such a negative impact on the children, early identification, prevention and treatment of substance use in families are crucial in preventing the intergenerational transmission of problems associated with parental substance abuse.

While the effects of maternal drinking after childbirth have been documented in various studies, it appears that substance use during pregnancy, both for fathers and mothers, has important clinical implications. Bailey and colleagues examined data from Seattle's Social Development Project, which included both men and women in the perinatal period. Their results showed that men's binge drinking and marijuana use were not reduced by their partner's pregnancy and/ or the advent of fatherhood. The conclusion of this study was that men's substance use was not affected by their partners' pregnancy and that the first few months postpartum may present a critical opportunity for substance use interventions. For Adam, the cocaine abuse began in pregnancy due to stress and escalated after Zoe's birth with added responsibilities and family duties. Had it continued without detection, it would have likely worsened with time. It is important to educate fathers about the impact of substance use on their child's development and on subsequent use behaviour of their partner. The only exception to Bailey et al.'s findings on substance use behaviour was with cigarette smoking in men. This was found to occur much less or actually decline significantly during the pregnancy of their partner. However, cigarette smoking returned rapidly to previous levels after the birth of the child. It could be assumed that this change in behaviour was found because the "second-hand smoke" could potentially affect the foetus, thereby modifying the father's behaviour, albeit temporarily.

The effects of addiction on parental involvement, especially the father's participation as the child grows up, have been studied by McMahon and colleagues. They investigated the status of 50 fathers who were attending methadone-maintenance treatment clinics and had fathered at least one child. The study's conclusion was interesting in that most fathers with substance use disorders wished to maintain contact and support their child and were interested in parenting-skills programmes. This is not surprising, as these fathers were already seeking help and thereby motivated to become better parents. This data thereby provided the evidence that although fathers were struggling with addiction, they did make attempts to be responsible parents in a socially accept-able manner. In the same study, however, men were most involved in the early fathering of their child, but their involvement decreased over time as their substance abuse continued and their relationship with the child's mother increased. This also correlated with diminished financial sup-port. It is therefore important to understand how negative experiences with a father or a father figure can contribute to a cross-generational deterioration of effective fathering. Adam felt abandoned by his father who was an alcoholic. Most of his life, Adam was angry at his father as he watched his mother being abused on a regular basis. He used to be anxious and moribund with fear when his father would come home drunk at night and ill-treat his mother. His own behav-iour with Daniella was beginning to resemble that of his father which ultimately scared him.

The association between maternal substance abuse and its effect on infants or young children has been studied more extensively than parental substance use and its impact on the child. Fathers provide much less direct care compared to mothers; however, with changing societal roles, hands-on fathers are becoming the norm rather than the exception. Therefore, the topic of how paternal alcohol use or abuse may influence the family dynamics, specifically that of the development of the child, is equally important to understand. Some investigators in the past have identified substance abuse as a specific risk factor for child abuse. Partner vio-lence, functioning of the parental dyad and parenting behav-iours are all modulated by substance-abusing fathers. Upon adulthood, individuals who were maltreated by their fathers often interact pathologically with their own families, includ-ing abuse not only towards their spouses but also towards their children. The National Longitudinal Alcohol Epidemiological Survey shows that approximately one in four children in the United States under the age of 18 lives with a family member who abuses alcohol. These children in turn are at risk for emotional and behavioural problems, and the likelihood of them perpetuating this violent behaviour in their own life is high. Therefore, it is critical to offer early intervention to prevent the deleterious effects of parental substance misuse on children. Daniella was made aware of the extent of Adam's struggle with substance abuse by his mother. She worried about the safety of the baby as well as her own security. When this realization dawned upon her, she took a decisive action to get help for Adam for the well-being of their family unit. Adam's mother further confided in Daniella that his paternal grandfather was an opium addict. The generational substance abuse pattern was clearly a risk factor for Adam. Environmental factors, specifically strain and pressure of child birth, were further determinants of increased susceptibilities for Adam who was already genetically predisposed.

Intimate Partner Violence and Substance Use Disorder

The co-occurrence of substance use and intimate partner violence is rather alarming in its frequency. There has been a fair amount of literature published on this phenomenon; some studies show that alcohol use and intimate partner violence (IPV) may be causally related, since direct disinhibition can lead to committing physical abuse. This was one of the main reasons in the case of Adam, why Daniella had to call 911. Sometimes cocaine intoxication and withdrawal symptoms can also lead to aggressive episodes. In those who abuse multiple substances at the same time and are withdrawing, any number of different outcomes may lead to IPV. IPV is a serious societal problem that must be addressed once it is established. This is especially prescient in new fathers where the safety of the baby is concerned as partner violence may also result in violence towards the baby. When the partner is intoxicated, whether male or female, the tragic consequences on a newborn baby are unpredictable. Many cases that come into child protection agencies are perpetuated by chronic substance use disorders and IPV. The prediction of whether specific substance use disorders or combinations of various disorders predict severe perpetration/victimization in males and females entering substance use treatment was studied by Kraanen and colleagues in 2014. They examined 1799 patients who were screened for IPV. In this particular study, they found that almost one third of the sample committed or experienced IPV in the past year. They found that alcohol use disorder combined with cannabis and/or cocaine disorder significantly predicted IPV perpetration in males compared to those with alcohol disorder alone. With females, they found that alcohol and cocaine abuse or dependence predicted both IPV and severe IPV perpetration. What is important to understand is that it is not always the female partner who is victimized. Often they can also be the perpetrators. However, in a postpartum situation, this is unlikely as the woman is normally busy with her newborn baby, sleep-deprived and struggling with exhaustion and lack of energy.

In a study by Reingle, it was found that IPV prevention and intervention efforts should account for the fact that in any IPV episode, the roles of victim and perpetrator may not be clearly discernible. They suggested that prevention and intervention strategies should target modifiable risk factors and address mental health issues in general. Gender-specific programming and culturally tailored components should focus on differential risk in subgroups. In the Reingle study, it appeared that African-American and Hispanic women were more likely to be victims. In another study, the link between alcohol abuse and male to female partner violence, as well as female to male partner violence, was studied. They analysed 50 independent studies. Their conclusion was that problem drinking is more likely to be linked with partner abuse than drinking per se and that alcohol consumption does likely contribute to increased partner violence. However, partner aggression is a multi-determined phenomenon with usually multiple risk factors requiring attention for effective intervention. It also appears from another study that couples that experience drinking-related social consequences are likely to experience higher levels of marital discord, fights and verbal aggression, placing them at a high risk for IPV. This study was done in 2002 by Cunradi and colleagues, where the association between male and female substance use problems and the risk of moderate to severe male IPV in general population samples was investigated. Another important link found in this study was that of high unemployment rates and intimate partner violence. Therefore, it is important to understand that there are several different factors that increase the risk for IPV in couples. Finally, the impact of IPV on young children had deleterious effects, both in the short and long term. One of the issues that Adam struggled with earlier in his life was watching the verbal altercations between his parents. Often, couples who engage in this type of interaction are unaware of the struggles their children will eventually have with regard to witnessing such behaviours at home. When Adam eventually got into therapy, he realized that he was essentially mimicking his father's behaviours by now being the aggressor and possibly the perpetrator in his relationship with Daniella.

The Effect of Paternal Substance Use on Children

The US Department of Health and Human Services estimates that between one- and two-thirds of child maltreatment cases involve some degree of substance use. The negative consequences can range from covert damage that is mild, i.e. difficulty in establishing trusting relationships with people or being overly emotionally responsible in relationships, to clear developmental damages, such as FAS. Lastly, children and adolescents of parents with SUD are often seen to be at higher risk for internalizing problems, such as depression and anxiety, as well as externalizing problems such as anger outbursts, aggression, impulsiveness and conduct disorder problems.

Studies also go to show that a parent with SUD is three times more likely to physically and sexually abuse their own child. Subsequently, many of these children are at a higher risk for being arrested as juveniles and going on to commit other violent crimes. Often, SUD in a parent can lead to long-term separation of the parent and child for a variety of reasons, which can negatively impact the growing child's ability to attach and regulate affect and can lead to trauma responses. These children are frequently maltreated and grow up in a poor physical, intellectual, social and emotional environment, often going on to develop their own substance abuse issues. In such individuals, it is important to approach treatment in a system-based manner with special attention to multigenerational trauma. This was an important aspect of Adam's treatment when he was in hospital. In his family, not only his father but also his grandfather had substance use issues.

Many children whose parents have SUD become "parentified children", i.e. the caretaker is unable to meet the developmental needs of the child, so the child begins to parent themselves and perhaps younger siblings earlier than what is developmentally appropriate. This is especially common in families that have a large number of siblings. Often, the child may also begin to parent the parent, which can lead to reversal of dependency needs. This can end up with blurring the healthy boundaries in the parent-child relationship. In particular, the child may have a lack of self-awareness as well as an over-awareness of other's needs.

Many studies show that parents' moodiness, forgetfulness and preoccupation can create a chaotic, unpredictable environment for their children. Often, children experience symptoms of anxiety, depression, fear, shame, guilt and loneliness. They become confused and angry and are at risk of developing every childhood disorder in the DSM, with an especially high risk of PTSD, eating disorders and mood and anxiety disorders. As a result, educational problems such as difficulties in focusing, thinking and learning are not infrequent in these children, as their basic survival needs are not being met.

It is important to understand that the treatment outcome in individuals with SUD is not going to be adequate if the impact of drinking or substance use on the whole family is not considered. The family system must be factored in to understanding the disease development, as well as its maintenance, and in successful treatment intervention. The earlier that one intervenes with these families, the better the eventual outcome for the whole family unit.

Fals-Stewart and colleagues examined the predictors of psychosocial adjustments of children living in households with parents in where the father was entering treatment for substance abuse and the effects of postnatal parental exposure. Half the children were exposed prenatally to illicit drugs. The researchers examined the variables of parents' sociodemographic characteristics, their dyadic adjustments, father's severity of substance abuse and the parents' psychological adjustments. The results showed that the younger, lower-income, dyadically distressed, physically violent parents had children with higher levels of psychosocial maladjustments. Additionally, father's higher frequency of substance use, higher psychological distress in both parents and a diagnosis of antisocial personality disorders in fathers were associated with higher paediatric symptom checklist scores. Moreover, male to female aggression had the strongest association with children's maladjustments. Therefore, the findings show that the children of substance abusers are at higher risk for developing alcohol and drug use problems, as well as other psychiatric disorders, if their parents have this history. It is therefore important to identify, modify and remove causative forces in their environment and help them to enhance their coping skills.

Parental training programmes to lessen abuse potential and increase the use of positive non-violent discipline strategies are recommended. Studies also show that programmes that promote school readiness and academic achievement for abused children improve child outcomes compared to those who do not get such treatment. This was investigated by researchers who examined the association between child abuse and neglect, substance abuse and physical health outcomes in children. They did a longitudinal study over 30 years where individuals were most recently interviewed in their mid-30s. They found that those with maltreatment histories more frequently reported lifetime alcohol problems and were at greater risk for substance use. In addition, these findings remained significant after controlling for general and childhood-associated economic status.

All the above studies reinforce the same messaging, which is that treating children of substance-abusing parents is an important, integral aspect of overall management. In the case of new fathers who are struggling with substance abuse issues, one must always be careful about whether or not the father is not being emotionally available to their children, maltreating their children or causing physical harm. In a recent study by Rossow, parental drinking was found to be statistically significantly associated with child harm outcome measures. Again, such an association goes to show that early intervention with parents is imperative in order to protect the children from violence in the present or perpetuating the psychopathology in the child and adolescent later in life. This can potentially prevent intergenerational trauma.

Recommendations: How Do You Intervene?

A pilot study examined the effects of the therapeutic intervention parenting skills with behavioural couples therapy (PSBCT) on substance use, parenting and relationship conflicts among fathers with alcohol use disorders. In this study, there were 30 male participants who filled out a variety of different screening scales. They had a history of drinking as well as drug use, and there was also evidence of relationship violence. These fathers received either individual psychotherapy/behavioural couples therapy or PSBCT. The results showed that those fathers who were involved in the PSBCT group did better compared to those who received the control treatments. This particular type of treatment also resulted in less involvement with child protective services. PSBCT also helped reduce drinking and relationship conflicts. The study concluded that the parenting skills and behavioural couples therapy was an effective modality of treatment for parents with substance use and relationship conflict issues. One of the findings from this study has particular relevance in the community, specifically the outcome showing that PSBCT helped reduce child protection agency involvement. This suggests a promising approach to reducing the risk of maltreatment in families where the father is identified as a substance user. Clearly, a larger study with a randomized design is needed to confirm the findings of the pilot study. In clinical practice, paternal psychiatric issues come to light too late. Most new mothers are busy with the baby and are not aware of the extent of father's substance use. It is not uncommon for new dads to drink excessively to deal with the stress of coping with the reality of sudden and unforeseen change in the couple's lifestyle. Often, the father's struggle with addiction becomes apparent when the child protection agency gets involved.

In a recent paper by Carroll in 2016, an interesting study using a variety of different available treatment modalities was described. In this study, participants were individuals who were seeking outpatient treatment for cocaine dependency. Researchers wanted to evaluate the extent to which the addition of disulfiram and contingency management (DCM) for adherence and abstinence, alone or in combination, was seen to enhance the effect of cognitive behaviour therapy (CBT) for cocaine disorders. Although CBT has strong evidence for its efficacy in the treatment of cocaine dependency, the evidence also suggests that this particular type of psychotherapy may produce better rates of relapse prevention when combined with pharmacotherapy and/or behaviour therapy. Disulfiram is a medication that has good evidence in the treatment of cocaine dependence. Therefore, in this double-blind study, 99 cocaine-dependent individuals were randomized to receive either disulfiram or a placebo, with or without contingency management (CM). All participants were already in treatment with CBT. The conclusion of the study was that disulfiram was not found to provide benefit as an adjunct treatment to CBT alone or CBT with CM. Secondly, CM was found to provide significantly better benefit as an adjunct treatment to CBT with or without the disulfiram. Therefore, the results of this study show that CM seems to be a promising adjunctive treatment for cocaine use disorders, especially in those individuals who are receiving CBT. It took a while for Adam to get into a right treatment facility to receive the appropriate treatment for his cocaine and alcohol abuse. Adam was away from Daniella and the baby for 4 months in a residential setting, during which time his mother moved into the couple's house to help with the baby. She provided support and hope to Daniella who was frightened and upset situation unfolded. However, Daniella was grateful for the care and back-up from her mother-in-law who was there for the baby unconditionally.

The popularity of mindfulness-based psychotherapy is also gaining momentum in the treatment of substance abuse disorders. Despite the availability of a variety of different treatments for substance abuse disorders, it appears that at the present time, none of them are completely satisfactory. This is because relapse rates following treatment still remain as high as 60%. Therefore, any novel modality of instituting effective treatment still remains an important goal. In this context, mindfulness-based interventions (or MBIs) have been increasingly suggested as potential intervention approaches. Mindfulness is currently conceptualized as a nonjudgemental, acceptance-based treatment following the key elements of Buddhist spiritual practices. In this type of therapy, there is a focus towards reducing associated distress leading to changes in one's thoughts and patterns and allowing the person to accept present moment experiences, as well as unpleasant feelings. Chiesa and Serretti recently did a review examining evidence for the efficacy of MBIs in substance use treatment. MBIs analysed included mindfulness-based relapse prevention (MBRP), dialectical behaviour therapy, acceptance and commitment therapy, spiritual self-schema therapy as well as different types of meditation. All together, they reviewed approximately 24 studies. The conclusion of this study was that overall, mindfulness-based intervention seemed to reduce the consumption and misuse of several substances including alcohol, cocaine, methamphetamines, marijuana, cigarette smoking and opioids to a significantly higher extent than several other types of active or inactive control treatments. Also, the study found that MBIs can improve several psychological outcomes associated with substance abuse and increase mindfulness levels.

Alcoholics Anonymous and Narcotics Anonymous (AA and NA) are important evidence-based interventions that have helped millions of people around the world with regard to dealing with their substance use issues. A study done by Pagano in 2013 investigated the 10-year cause and impact of AA and their long-term outcomes on 226 treatment-seeking alcoholics. They found that the importance of meeting attendance in AA-related groups led to long-term behavioural changes and recovery in general. It is known that AA is an effective clinical and public health ally that aids addiction recovery through mobilization of mechanisms similar to those in formal treatment but is able to do so for free over the long term in the communities where participants live. Therefore, this method of treatment continues to be useful in bringing about behavioural changes in individuals. When looking at the efficacy of AA without self-selection bias, studies have shown that the intervention is helpful because the therapeutic process includes social support for healthy behavioural change, the availability of role models, insulation of hope and practical skill teaching.

Take-Home Messages

1. It is important to conduct screening assessments for potential substance use when seeing a couple, both in mothers and fathers.

2. Comorbidity of substance abuse and other psychiatric conditions is frequently encountered in clinical practice
3. Substance abuse and intimate partner violence are highly linked phenomena with extremely detrimental outcomes.
4. Men, children of alcoholics and those with sensation-seeking behaviours, low levels of planning, impulsive behaviours or coping techniques and/or neurobehavioural inhibition are more likely to abuse substances.
5. Paternal substance use has implications that are intergenerational, especially for children during their developmental period.
6. Over and above traditional treatments of the 12-step programme for alcohol and drug use, and/or hospitalization where necessary, there are a variety of modern treatments that include mindfulness psychotherapy, cognitive behaviour therapy and contingency management, parenting-skills training and couples therapy.

References

1. American Psychiatric Association. Diagnostic and statistical manual of mental disorders (DSM-5®). Arlington: American Psychiatric Pub; 2013.
2. Bailey JA, Hill KG, Hawkins JD, et al. Men's and women's patterns of substance use around pregnancy. Birth. 2008;35(1):50–9.
3. Brems C, Johnson ME, Neal D, et al. Childhood abuse history and substance use among men and women receiving detoxification services. Am J Drug Alcohol Abuse. 2004;30(4):799–821.
4. Brenner H, Mielck A. The role of childbirth in smoking cessation. Prev Med. 1992;22(2):225–36.
5. Brook JS, Zhang C, Rubenstone E, et al. Comorbid trajectories of substance use as predictors of antisocial personality disorder, major depressive episode, and generalized anxiety disorder. Addict Behav. 2016;62:114–21.
6. Carroll KM, Nich C, Petry NM, et al. A randomized factorial trial of disulfiram and contingency management to enhance cognitive behavioral therapy for cocaine dependence. Drug Alcohol Depend. 2016;160:135–42.

7. Chen LY, Strain EC, Crum RM, Mojtabai R. Gender differences in substance abuse treatment and barriers to care among persons with substance use disorders with and without comorbid major depression. J Addict Med. 2013;7(5):325.

8. Chiesa A, Serretti A. Are mindfulness-based interventions effective for substance use disorders? A systematic review of the evidence. Subst Use Misuse. 2014;49(5):492–512.

9. Christmon K, Luckey I. Is early fatherhood associated with alcohol and other drug use? J Subst Abus Treat. 1994;6(3):337–43.

10. Cunradi CB, Caetano R, Schafer J. Alcohol-related problems, drug use, and male intimate partner violence severity among US couples. Alcohol Clin Exp Res. 2002;26(4):493–500.

11. Duckworth AL, Chertok IR. Review of perinatal partner-focused smoking cessation interventions. MCN Am J Matern Child Nurs. 2012;37(3):174–81.

12. Emmerik-van Oortmerssen K, Glind G, Koeter MW. Psychiatric comorbidity in treatment-seeking substance use disorder patients with and without attention deficit hyperactivity disorder: results of the IASP study. Addiction. 2014;109(2):262–72.

13. Fals-Stewart W, Kelley ML, Cooke CG, et al. Predictors of the psychosocial adjustment of children living in households of parents in which fathers abuse drugs: the effects of postnatal parental exposure. Addict Behav. 2003;28(6):1013–31.

14. Fergusson DM, Boden JM, Horwood LJ. Transition to parenthood and substance use disorders: findings from a 30-year longitudinal study. Drug Alcohol Depend. 2012;125(3):295–300.

15. Foran HM, O'Leary KD. Alcohol and intimate partner violence: a meta-analytic review. Clin Psychol Rev. 2008;28(7):1222–34.

16. Garrusi S, Amirkafi A, Garrusi B. Experiences of drug dependent fathers in relation with their children: a qualitative study. Addict Health. 2011;3(1–2):29.

17. Grant BF, Stinson FS, Dawson DA, et al. Prevalence and co-occurrence of substance use disorders and independent mood and anxiety disorders: results from the national epidemiologic survey on alcohol and related conditions. Arch Gen Psychiatry. 2004;61(8):807–16.

18. Hasin DS, Stinson FS, Ogburn E, et al. Prevalence, correlates, disability, and comorbidity of DSM-IV alcohol abuse and dependence in the United States: results from the National Epidemiologic Survey on Alcohol and Related Conditions. Arch Gen Psychiatry. 2007;64(7):830–42.

19. Hoffmann JP, Cerbone FG. Parental substance use disorder and the risk of adolescent drug abuse: an event history analysis. Drug Alcohol Depend. 2002;66(3):255–64.
20. Herrenkohl TI, Hong S, Klika JB, Herrenkohl RC, Russo MJ. Developmental impacts of child abuse and neglect related to adult mental health, substance use, and physical health. J Fam Violence 2013;28:1–9.
21. Humphreys K, Blodgett JC, Wagner TH. Estimating the efficacy of Alcoholics Anonymous without self-selection bias: an instrumental variables re-analysis of randomized clinical trials. Alcohol Clin Exp Res. 2014;38(11):2688–94.
22. Jääskeläinen M, Holmila M, Notkola IL, et al. Mental disorders and harmful substance use in children of substance abusing parents: a longitudinal register-based study on a complete birth cohort born in 1991. Drug Alcohol Rev. 2016;35(6):728–40.
23. Kelly JF. Is Alcoholics Anonymous religious, spiritual, neither? Findings from 25 years of mechanisms of behavior change research. Addiction. 2017;112(6):929–36.
24. Kelley ML, Fals-Stewart W. Psychiatric disorders of children living with drug-abusing, alcohol-abusing, and non–substance-abusing fathers. J Am Acad Child Adolesc Psychiatry. 2004;43(5):621–8.
25. Klostermann KC, Fals-Stewart W. Intimate partner violence and alcohol use: exploring the role of drinking in partner violence and its implications for intervention. Aggress Violent Behav. 2006;11(6):587–97.
26. Kraanen FL, Vedel E, Scholing A, et al. Prediction of intimate partner violence by type of substance use disorder. J Subst Abus Treat. 2014;46(4):532–9.
27. Lam WK, Fals-Stewart W, Kelley ML. Parent training with behavioral couples therapy for fathers' alcohol abuse: effects on substance use, parental relationship, parenting, and CPS involvement. Child Maltreat. 2009;14(3):243–54.
28. Lander L, Howsare J, Byrne M. The impact of substance use disorders on families and children: from theory to practice. Soc Work Public Health. 2013;28(3–4):194–205.
29. McMahon TJ, Winkel JD, Suchman NE, et al. Drug-abusing fathers: patterns of pair bonding, reproduction, and paternal involvement. J Subst Abus Treat. 2007;33(3):295–302.
30. McCrory EJ, Mayes L. Understanding addiction as a developmental disorder: an argument for a developmentally informed multilevel approach. Curr Addict Rep. 2015;2(4):326–30.

31. Merline AC, O'Malley PM, Schulenberg JE, et al. Substance use among adults 35 years of age: prevalence, adulthood predictors, and impact of adolescent substance use. Am J Public Health. 2004;94(1):96–102.

32. Moss HB, Clark DB, Kirisci L. Timing of paternal substance use disorder cessation and effects on problem behaviors in sons. Am J Addict. 1997;6(1):30–7.

33. Pagano ME, White WL, Kelly JF, et al. The 10-year course of Alcoholics Anonymous participation and long-term outcomes: a follow-up study of outpatient subjects in Project MATCH. Subst Abuse. 2013;34(1):51–9.

34. Pelham WE Jr, Lang AR. Can your children drive you to drink. Alcohol Res Health. 1999;23(4):292–8.

35. Reingle JM, Jennings WG, Connell NM, et al. On the pervasiveness of event-specific alcohol use, general substance use, and mental health problems as risk factors for intimate partner violence. J Interpers Violence. 2014;29(16):2951–70.

36. Rohsenow DJ, Monti PM, Martin RA, et al. Brief coping skills treatment for cocaine abuse: 12-month substance use outcomes. J Consult Clin Psychol. 2000;68(3):515.

37. Rossow I, Felix L, Keating P, et al. Parental drinking and adverse outcomes in children: a scoping review of cohort studies. Drug Alcohol Rev. 2016;35(4):397–405.

38. Sinha R. How does stress increase risk of drug abuse and relapse? Psychopharmacology. 2001;158(4):343–59.

39. Smith DK, Johnson AB, Pears KC, et al. Child maltreat and foster care: unpacking the effects of prenatal and postnatal parental substance use. Child Maltreat. 2007;12(2):150–60.

40. Stone AL, Becker LG, Huber AM, et al. Review of risk and protective factors of substance use and problem use in emerging adulthood. Addict Behav Rep. 2012;37(7):747–75.

41. Walitzer KS, Dearing RL. Gender differences in alcohol and substance use relapse. Clin Psychol Rev. 2006;26(2):128–48.

Chapter 9
New Fathers with Narcissistic Personality Disorders: When Dad Becomes Too Self-Absorbed

---

Dad's Story: The Story of a Selfish Dad

Michael and Jessie met at the university, a combination of "beauty and brains." The winner of a local beauty pageant, Jessie excelled in sports and held a rowing scholarship. Michael was a charming, talented, determined young man on a basketball scholarship; he eventually became an international basketball player. Jessie and Michael were perfect match, the envy of many friends and had an ideal marriage until their first baby was born. A prolonged, traumatic labour led to Jessie's development of generalized anxiety disorder. After numerous phone calls and pleading requests from Jessie's family, Michael flew home from Miami in the middle of his basketball season. He could neither comprehend nor come to terms with her struggle or her cry for help. Michael was unable to be empathetic or understanding of Jessie's needs. Preoccupied with a sense of self-importance, Michael was fixated on his success and accomplishments. He loved the admiration that came with being a super-

(continued)

© Springer International Publishing AG 2018　　　　167
S.K. Misri, *Paternal Postnatal Psychiatric Illnesses*,
https://doi.org/10.1007/978-3-319-68249-5_9

hero and was not particularly concerned about being a good partner or father. He believed that Jessie's illness reflected poorly on him. Michael became totally self-absorbed; he picked fights and became increasingly arrogant with the passage of time. His perception of being "special" and his demand for constant attention led to irreconcilable differences in their marriage. Reluctantly, Michael agreed to seek marital therapy in order to salvage his public image.

Michael's diagnosis of narcissistic personality disorder emerged during their sessions with the therapist. The therapist's diagnosis of narcissistic personality disorder came as a surprise to Michael. The essential features of this disorder are ongoing or pervasive patterns of self-admiration and a sense of grandiosity, beginning in early adulthood. In understanding why he developed these personality traits, he had to come to grips with the environment of growing up with his parents' specific styles of parenting, which obviously affected him. Reflecting on his own childhood, Michael realized there were a lot of authoritarian parenting styles that he was exposed to from his own father, who was an athlete himself. However, his father did not achieve the same level of recognition as Michael and saw himself as a failure as a result. In his own way, Michael's father then lived through Michael to fulfil his own sense of self-gratification, thereby increasing the burden on the expectations of Michael as he grew up. In some sense, Michael felt that he was robbed of his childhood because the pressure to perform was "on" from a very early age. Adding to this, he remembered that his mother, who was a strict high school teacher, was not a very loving parent. His mother was absent much of the time, and even when she was present, she was not very engaging. Overall Michael felt quite neglected by both of his parents.

Although it was important for Michael to understand how he developed these characteristics growing up, it was

(continued)

not easy to change his interpersonal way of communicating with Jessie. The problem in the marriage that was particularly difficult for her to handle was his grandiose sense of self-importance. Because he was such a famous athlete and had a lot of people admiring him, asking him for his autograph and wanting to pose for photographs with him, he lived an isolated life away from Jessie, and now the newborn baby, in a world completely different than most people. He put a lot of his own sense of identity in these attributes and valued this sort of existence which he repeatedly talked about in therapy. Often, his judgment of his own accomplishments was the ongoing awards and hefty compensation for his excellent skills that he displayed. However, these same attributes did not serve him well in his personal life. In fact, his idealized sense of self, success, power and privilege of his life compared to others came back to haunt him. He continued to ruminate while he was at home in the midst of therapy, sorting out his new role as a father. He missed his old life and definitely had to make a choice between being at home with Jessie in an "ordinary life" versus the very privileged lifestyle he had away from his family. Michael always wanted to be the best and the top of his game, no matter what he did outside of his family constellation, and, therefore, after a year of trying to be a reasonable partner and a good father, the end result was that Michael and Jessie decided to go their separate ways.

Michael's sense of self-esteem was very fragile. At home, he did not have the usual fanfare and was not greeted with the kind of reverence that he was used to in his professional and social life. The fact that Jessie needed and wanted more from him, especially in the context of her own anxiety and mood issues and taking on the role of a new mother, meant that he was not able to meet her needs as well. Another interesting characteristic of a lot of personality-disordered people is that their romantic relationships will only work for them if there is some sense of

(continued)

enhancement of their self-esteem and if the relationship in some way advances their own purpose. None of these were applicable now in the new life that they had chosen for themselves, which was obviously not what Michael had anticipated earlier or had sought out. The other issue was his lack of empathy generally in their relationship, which became a critical factor. This trait was especially noticeable when Jessie invited her parents to come and help her, as she was desperate to get extra help with the baby. A couple of times, her mother did remark on this specific issue of Michael's lack of feelings for others, which also included Jessie's parents and his total lack of concern for the welfare of anybody other than himself. The impatience, short fuse and angry outbursts did not have a positive effect on their relationship either. In fact, they caused more of a rift, especially when his behaviour would change completely in the presence of strangers, in front of whom he would be boasting about his lifetime achievements, whereas in the privacy of their home, with Jessie and his extended family, he would be completely different. The lack of emotional sensitivity and the ongoing coldness eventually resulted in the break-up of this relationship.

DSM-5 Diagnosis

Narcissistic Personality Disorder (NPD)

A pervasive pattern of grandiosity, need for admiration and lack of empathy beginning in early childhood and present in a variety of contexts as indicated by five or more of the following:

1. *Has a grandiose sense of self-importance*
2. *Is preoccupied with fantasies of unlimited success, power, brilliance, beauty or ideal love*
3. *Believes that he or she is "special and unique" and can only be understood by, or should associate with, other "special or high-status" people*

4. *Requires excessive admiration*
5. *Has a sense of entitlement*
6. *Is interpersonally exploitative*
7. *Lacks empathy: Is unwilling to recognize or identify with the feelings and needs of others*
8. *Is often envious of others, believes that others are envious of him or her and shows arrogant, haughty behaviours or attitudes*

Review of the Disorder

Epidemiology

Prevalence estimates for narcissistic personality disorder, based on the DSM-4 definition, range anywhere between 0% and 6.2% in community samples. Of those, it appears that there are also gender-related diagnostic differences between personality disorders. For instance, of those diagnosed with narcissistic personality disorder, about 50–75% were identified to be male. An earlier paper by Phillipson and colleagues published in 1985 aimed to investigate the gender bias in diagnosis and etiological explanation of narcissistic personality disorder. In this paper, the researchers found that men are more likely to display feelings of grandiosity and extreme self-centredness. Female narcissists appear to see romantic partners as part of their self and ego, while males typically used their female love partners as self-esteem boosts, as Michael did in his own life.

With regard to the prevalence of NPD in the community, Dhawan and colleagues did a comparison in 2009 of the prevalence rate between clinical and non-clinical samples by using structured clinical interviews. The results of this specific study showed that the prevalence rates existent in the clinical samples varied from 2.3% to 35.7%, a very large range in variation, whereas the low prevalence rate in the community sample was found to have a wide range of 0–6.2%, with a mean prevalence rate of 1.06%. Clearly, this big difference in the two types of samples needs to be studied further; however, it appears that as far as narcissistic personality disorder is concerned, by the time a person is referred to a specialist by the family physician or other agencies that refer them for treatment, the individual has clearly been impaired in some way which requires them to seek help from a specialist. On the other hand, those who mostly exhibit the positive attributes of such a personality, where the person does not behave in an impaired manner, may or may not seek help or get the attention of researchers. This may potentially explain why there is such a difference in the prevalence rates of these two samples. From a clinical point of view, the personality disorder of narcissism is important to recognize and treat, because with time the prognosis worsens and the increased possibility of suicidality in such individuals is always a concern. The vulnerability to suicidal behaviour was described by Heisel. Often, there is an overlapping between other types of personality disorders and NPD. For instance, borderline and histrionic personality disorders have been found to overlap with the narcissistic personality. Persons with histrionic personality disorders are often self-dramatizing, superfluously gregarious, seductive, shallow and exhibitionistic. The feature of demanding attention is common to both NPD and those with histrionic features. People with borderline personality disorder are often self-destructive and show self-damaging behaviours, and impulsivity is a central feature of this particular personality disorder. In particular, erratic temper tantrums and emotional instability are striking features of those with borderline personality disorder. Often these disorders are under the umbrella of Cluster B personality disorders, which also includes antisocial personality disorders. All of these disorders by and large are difficult to treat; however, giving them a diagnostic classification often makes treatment easier. For instance, narcissism is typically treated with psychosocial interventions, whereas approaches for borderline personality disorder include dialectical behaviour therapy (or DBT). Histrionic personality disorder, which is often associated with somatic symptom disorder, tends to warrant treatment with psychoeducation, psychodynamic therapy and, most commonly, supportive psychotherapy in order to deal with their dependency needs.

Risk Factors

Research has suggested that some types of parental child-rearing behaviours may be associated with risk for offspring personality disorder. In a research by Johnson and colleagues, they used a community-based sample of 593 families and their children and studied them longitudinally from age 6 to age 33. They were seen during adolescence, around age 14–16 and then around age 22. In this study, the researchers found that low parental nurturing and aversive parental behaviours during child rearing may be associated with elevated risk for personality disorders in the offspring. This is of importance especially given that early intervention after a diagnosis is made can potentially alter the course of the maladaptive parental patterns, which may have positive effects on the children in the long term. Some types of parenting practices such as harsh punishment or lack of affection or nurturing may be associated with the risk of personality disorders that can persist into adulthood. Therefore, educating parents about these problematic parental styles may be of value. Early intervention can also promote improved communication and increase warmth and nurturing, thereby ensuring a positive sense of self-esteem and development in the child. It appears in this study that both maternal behaviours and problematic paternal communication patterns were associated with elevated risk in the offspring.

A number of different studies have shown how children of narcissistic parents turn out in their own lives. The therapist also raised the possibility in treating Michael that his own parents may have had some tendencies towards narcissism themselves. A paper by Rappoport published in 2005 concluded that being a child of narcissistic parents may result in either identification with the parents, which is what Michael did; compliance, which is also what he showed all throughout his teenage years and early adulthood; or finally rebellion, a behaviour that he was familiar with during his marriage to Jessie. Dr. Rappoport believes that, in particular, children of narcissistic parents also engage in a phenomenon called co-narcissism. Co-narcissism is also described as a phenomenon very close to co-alcoholism in that it occurs in a person who has adapted to the life of narcissistic people, in this case with Michael, it was his own parents, and unconsciously collaborating with these individuals and somehow taking on the problems of their narcissism in his own life.

Narcissism is a personality form that resembles addiction to self-esteem. Typically, this kind of pattern can emerge well before adulthood. Essentially, narcissism is seen as an ongoing personality process organized around the goal of creating and maintaining grandiose self-abuse. In narcissism, there is a continuous need for aggrandizement from others. Very little is known about its aetiology and development. Those with NPD tend to value other people only when they can help them achieve their own self-centred goals. This is an important characteristic of NPD individuals, as they are generally self-absorbed extroverts who tend to block negative experiences from their conscious awareness. One of the most influential models of narcissism is the dynamic self-regulatory processing model. In this model, it appears that on an interpersonal level, the narcissist tends to mould their social interaction by trying to establish their own superiority. They tend to crave attention, and if they do not get this sort of admiration, they can become quite aggressive. These individuals always want to feel good about themselves and are seeking ways to achieve that goal.

Specific maladaptive socializing experiences combined with biologically based temperamental traits are thought to be possible factors responsible for the development of narcissism. These socializing experiences refer to parental evaluation of the child. For instance, the parent can be over-indulgent, can be cold or have high expectations. These factors can play a role in the development of narcissism. The way that children react to positive or negative stimuli is often referred to in the literature as approach and/or avoidance temperament, which is responsible for the child's behaviour. Although little or nothing is known about how narcissism really develops in a person's life, it rarely manifests itself before the age of 8, and often it emerges in late childhood.

Temperamental influence is also an important aspect of the emergence of narcissism, and clearly more studies need to take place to examine the interplay between genes and environment. It is also important to identify what sort of factors influence this disorder to persist over time and how we can minimize the burden such a disorder places on others. For instance, narcissistic injury is a common result of the splitting of the different mechanisms that most significantly predict NPD. The common defence mechanisms that a person with narcissism uses are projection, intellectualization, omnipotence, splitting others images, devaluation, rationalization, denial, acting out, passive aggression and splitting of self-images. Frequently, these types of defences are also present in those with antisocial personality disorder. Individuals with NPD are often sensitive and respond in a highly aggressive or explosive way, which can be difficult for the family or community to deal with. In a paper by Holtzman, the narcissistic behaviours of 80 undergraduate students were investigated in a naturalistic setting. They found that narcissism was positively correlated with disagreeable acts, greater sexual language use and more exploitativeness and entitlement in general. They concluded that narcissists displayed distinct behaviours in their everyday lives and they tended to be impulsive and seek short-term gains. Additionally, there appeared to be a link between narcissism and short-term promiscuous sexual strategy.

A recent study by Luchner explored whether there is a relationship between competitive individuals and overt and covert narcissism. The study showed that high levels of narcissism were present in the sample of over 300 undergraduate students who were surveyed for the specific desire to be hyper-competitive. In addition, it was found that there was a positive relationship between overt and covert narcissism with competitiveness and hyper-competitiveness, respectively. Also, the authors found that those who were covertly narcissistic avoided conflicts and were over-reactive to unfulfilled expectations. Competitiveness present among athletes, bodybuilders and certain types of university students such as those studying psychology is also an interesting way of examining narcissism in this population. Bodybuilders are generally found to be more narcissistic compared to athletes and psychology students, and men and masculine groups also tend to have higher levels of narcissism than women or feminine groups. Interestingly enough, there also appears to be a correlation between anabolic steroid use and higher entitlement and exploitative factors in those weight lifters and bodybuilders who use this substance. A connection was found to exist between narcissism and steroid use in a study by Carroll of 36 male weight lifters who were on steroids. However, it was not clear if narcissism was a cause or an effect of the steroid use. In a recent study, researchers from Bishop's University investigated university football players and narcissistic personality traits and whether or not the concept of narcissism in football players was a stereotype versus a reality. They found that other athletes perceived football players as more narcissistic. Presumably this was because football players were often seen as demanding privileges for themselves around the campus and also saw narcissism as an advantage, i.e. that they were able to intimidate others with these kinds of personality traits. These findings again point towards some of the difficulties that Jessie had in her ability to cope with the personality traits that Michael displayed during their relationship and further goes to emphasize the need for early intervention and treatment.

Correlation between depression and narcissism has been described in the analytic literature in psychiatry. A study was done by Shona Tritt and her colleagues, who wanted to study the link between depression and narcissism assessed depressive temperament and its relationship to narcissistic personality disorder (NPD) in 228 university students. A number of different measures that were administered included narcissistic personality inventory, temperament evaluation and a schedule for fatigue and anergia. The researchers made an interesting connection between two different components of pathological narcissistic personality traits and affect. The authors looked at grandiosity and vulnerability and their relationship to negative affect when the narcissistic needs were not met. In this study, it was noted that depression temperament was associated with narcissistic disturbance, especially in relation to avoiding the narcissistic injury. Narcissistic injury generally has to do with their perception of self-image. Some researchers in the past have seen that this could be interpreted as a defence against possible depression. Other traits such as entitlement and exploitative tendencies are positively related to depression. In the case of Michael, the anxiety traits that were evident during therapy were noted to be associated with a sense of entitlement. Often, people with this type of disorder are vulnerable and that trait in itself is seen as being related to depressive risk in the future. Overall, it appears that certain vulnerable and maladaptive narcissistic traits appear to be positively associated with depressive traits. In addition to depressive temperaments, there are other conditions such as cyclothymic personality and anxiousness and hyperthymic temperaments that are seen to contribute to the development of narcissistic personality. It is important to find ways to help patients with depressive temperament to develop self-esteem that is less contingent upon recognition from others. It also requires focus with respect to how to deal with these individuals' interpersonal coldness, their reactivity to certain situations and social avoidance. Further studies are needed to be done in this area in order to understand these connections in depth.

It appears that with Michael, his grandiose type of traits that he had exhibited through most of his adolescence and adult years, as suggested by Tritt and other researchers made him more vulnerable. He used avoidance as a means to deal with a lot of his tension and anxiety. In therapy, his increased level of intrapsychic anxiety, which was part and parcel of his depression, made him more vulnerable; he was unable to cope with the reality of fatherhood. The birth of the baby, in Michael's case, was seen as "injury" for him rather than a welcome addition to his family. A lot of the time, narcissistic individuals just want adulation for themselves; they crave for affection, love and admiration in a selfish way. They do not want to share the attention with anybody else. Michael could not handle sharing his wife's affection with the new baby.

NPD and how it relates to other psychiatric conditions have not been studied with regard to new fathers. Most of the studies on comorbidity between narcissistic personality disorder and psychiatric manifestations have involved the general population. With regard to the association between substance dependence disorders and personality disorders in general, it appears that there is a strong correlation to alcohol, drugs and tobacco. Personality disorders, by definition, constitute patterns of inner experiences and behaviours that are inflexible and pervasive over time. They usually begin in early adolescence or early adulthood and, in general, appear to be associated with anxiety and mood disorders. These are the individuals who are basically more prone to developing substance use when they are in their adulthood. Because many individuals with personality disorders experience emotional dysregulation as well as impulse problems, they appear to be more vulnerable to overuse of any types of substances, eventually developing dependence on them. Trull and colleagues showed that any type of personality disorder diagnosis had over 12 times more risk of developing lifetime diagnosis of drug dependence than those without a personality disorder diagnosis. Studies also show that individuals with personality disorders endorse more perceived stress and less interpersonal support, and it has also been reported that they have higher rates of suicidal behaviours, legal troubles and significantly higher rates of occupational, romantic and interpersonal problems over the preceding years.

When it comes to the narcissistic personality, it appears that bipolar 1 and GAD are more correlated to this type of personality and gender differences are worth noting as antisocial and narcissistic personality disorders appeared to be more significant in men compared to women. In a study done by Stinson and colleagues, they showed that narcissistic personality disorder was more prevalent among black men and women, as well as those of Hispanic descent and those who were separated, divorced, widowed or never-married adults.

The method used in this particular study was face-to-face interviews with over 34,000 adults who participated in the National Epidemiologic Survey on alcohol and related disorders. The conclusion of this study was that narcissistic personality disorder was prevalent in the general US population and was associated with a considerable disability in men and that the rates of disability actually did exceed those of women. This is an interesting study from the point of view of how expression of narcissism in men could impact their functionality over their lifetime. In this particular study, narcissism was seen to be highly correlated to a variety of different psychiatric conditions, which included not just substance use but also panic disorder, agoraphobia and bipolar 1 disorder as well. There appears to be a propensity of men with narcissistic personality disorder to self-medicate in order to maintain a sense of grandiosity, as they have fragile self-esteem. Their sense of omnipotence can be maintained if they use substances in order to escape from the reality of their situation. They also deal with their feelings of depression and guilt or dysthymia that may be associated with their sense of grandiosity.

Although there were issues with his growing up, Michael did perceive his family to be supportive of him. This served as a protective factor; he was able to engage in therapy in a more positive manner; he was not in trouble with the law; he did not show any suicidal behaviours and the depressive symptoms were not severe enough to need medication therapy. With psychotherapy alone, he responded well to treating many of these temperamental traits. Michael and Jessie worked really hard in therapy with regard to their interpersonal relationship, as well as issues pertaining to his narcissism. What became clear was that Michael, unfortunately, was not able to handle the role of being a new father, and Jessie was really concerned about its impact on their child. When it became clear that he was not willing to make any changes, unfortunately they decided to live separately and pursue growth individually as well as continue to maintain a cordial relationship for the sake of their child.

Comorbidity

Correlation between depression and narcissism has been described in the analytic literature in psychiatry. A study was done by Shona Tritt and her colleagues, who wanted to study the link between depression and narcissism assessed depressive temperament and its relationship to narcissistic personality disorder (NPD) in 228 university students. A number of different measures that were administered included narcissistic personality inventory, temperament evaluation and a schedule for fatigue and anergia. The researchers made an interesting connection between two different components of pathological narcissistic personality traits and affect. The authors looked at grandiosity and vulnerability and their relationship to negative affect when the narcissistic needs were not met. In this study, it was noted that depression temperament was associated with narcissistic disturbance, especially in relation to avoiding the narcissistic injury. Narcissistic injury generally has to do with their perception of self-image. Some researchers in the past have seen that this could be interpreted as a defence against possible depression. Other traits such as entitlement and exploitative tendencies are positively related to depression. In the case of Michael, the anxiety traits that were evident during therapy were noted to be associated with a sense of entitlement. Often, people with this type of disorder are vulnerable and that trait in itself is seen as being related to depressive risk in the future. Overall, it appears that certain vulnerable and maladaptive narcissistic traits appear to be positively associated with depressive traits. In addition to depressive temperaments, there are other conditions such as cyclothymic personality and anxiousness and hyperthymic temperaments that are seen to contribute to the development of narcissistic personality. It is important to find ways to help patients with depressive temperament to develop self-esteem that is less contingent upon recognition from others. It also requires focus with respect to how to deal with these individuals' interpersonal coldness, reactivity to certain situations and social avoidance. Further studies are needed to be done in this area in order to understand these connections in depth.

It appears that with Michael, his grandiose type of traits that he had exhibited through most of his adolescence and adult years, as suggested by Tritt and other researchers, made him more vulnerable. He used avoidance as a means to deal with a lot of his tension and anxiety. In therapy, his increased level of intrapsychic anxiety, which was part and parcel of his depression, made him more vulnerable; he was unable to cope with the reality of fatherhood. The birth of the baby, in Michael's case, was seen as "injury" for him rather than a welcome addition to his family. A lot of the time, narcissistic individuals just want adulation for themselves; they crave for affection, love and admiration in a selfish way. They do not want to share the attention with anybody else. Michael could not handle sharing his wife's affection with the new baby.

NPD and how it relates to other psychiatric conditions have not been studied with regard to new fathers. Most of the studies on comorbidity between narcissistic personality disorder and psychiatric manifestations have involved the general population. With regard to the association between substance dependence disorders and personality disorders in general, it appears that there is a strong correlation to alcohol, drugs and tobacco. Personality disorders, by definition, constitute patterns of inner experiences and behaviours that are inflexible and pervasive over time. They usually begin in early adolescence or early adulthood and, in general, appear to be associated with anxiety and mood disorders. These are the individuals who are basically more prone to developing substance use when they are in their adulthood. Because many individuals with personality disorders experience emotional dysregulation as well as impulse problems, they appear to be more vulnerable to overuse of any types of substances, eventually developing dependence on them. Trull and colleagues showed that any type of personality disorder diagnosis had over 12 times more risk of developing lifetime diagnosis of drug dependence than those without a personality disorder diagnosis. Studies also show that individuals with personality disorders endorse more perceived stress and less interpersonal support, and it has also been reported that they have higher rates of suicidal behaviours, legal troubles and significantly higher rates of occupational, romantic and interpersonal problems over the preceding years.

When it comes to the narcissistic personality, it appears that bipolar 1 and GAD are more correlated to this type of personality. Additionally, gender differences are worth noting as antisocial and narcissistic personality disorders appeared to be more significant in men compared to women. In a study done by Stinson and colleagues, they showed that narcissistic personality disorder was more prevalent among black men and women, as well as those of Hispanic descent and those who were separated, divorced, widowed or never-married adults. The method used in this particular study was face-to-face interviews with over 34,000 adults who participated in the National Epidemiologic Survey on alcohol and related disorders. The conclusion of this study was that narcissistic personality disorder was prevalent in the general US population and was associated with a considerable disability in men and that the rates of disability actually did exceed those of women. This is an interesting study from the point of view of how expression of narcissism in men could impact their functionality over their lifetime. In this particular study, narcissism was seen to be highly correlated to a variety of different psychiatric conditions, which included not just substance use but also panic disorder, agoraphobia and bipolar 1 disorder as well. There appears to be a propensity of men with narcissistic personality disorder to self-medicate in order to maintain a sense of grandiosity, as they have fragile self-esteem. Their sense of omnipotence can be maintained if they use substances in order to escape from the reality of their situation. They also deal with their feelings of depression and guilt or dysthymia that may be associated with their sense of grandiosity.

Although there were issues with his growing up, Michael did perceive his family to be supportive of him. This served as a protective factor; he was able to engage in therapy in a more positive manner; he was not in trouble with the law; he did not show any suicidal behaviours and the depressive symptoms were not severe enough to need medication therapy. With psychotherapy alone, he responded well to treating many of these temperamental traits. Michael and Jessie worked really hard in therapy with regard to their interpersonal relationship, as well as issues pertaining to his narcissism. What became clear was that Michael, unfortunately, was not able to handle the role of being a new father, and Jessie was really concerned about its impact on their child. When it became clear that he was not willing to make any changes, unfortunately they decided to live separately and pursue growth individually as well as continue to maintain a cordial relationship for the sake of their child.

Treatment Recommendations: How Do You Intervene?

With regard to treatment, by and large narcissists fail to form attachments, and thus the use of psychotherapy can be limited. They also form attachments through aloofness, and this can be difficult in a patient/therapist relationship. However, generally, integrative models of therapy are recommended depending on how well the patient is able to tolerate anxiety, control impulses and develop meaningful relationships. Typically, the goal of therapy for those with narcissistic personality disorder is to develop empathy and focus on impulse control. Group therapy treatments can be problematic, but they have been found to be useful by some researchers, as indicated by Kraus and Reynolds. Conjoined marital therapy has also been found to be useful. A 2015 article in the *American Journal of Psychiatry* highlights that the effectiveness of psychotherapy and/or pharmacotherapy in the treatment of narcissistic personality disorder has not been investigated systematically. Therefore, appropriate practice guidelines for this disorder have yet to be formulated.

It appears that psychopharmacological intervention is generally appropriate when certain symptoms are seen. Regardless of the severity, the grandiosity and defensiveness which characterize this personality disorder make any form of engagement in a psychotherapeutic alliance difficult. The current treatment recommendations are presently based largely on clinical experiences and different treatment approaches based on psychodynamic formulation. While large-scale, properly conducted studies do not exist, individual case reports suggest that psychotherapeutic treatments can be effective for some patients but not for all. In an article by Caligor and her colleagues, recommendation is made for empirically supported treatments for borderline personality disorder which can be adapted for NPD. In particular, these researchers recommend mentalization-based therapy, transference-focused psychotherapy and schema-focused cognitive therapy. These three treatments target some of the underlying features of narcissistic personality disorder. In addition, DBT or dialectical behaviour therapy is another option if there is comorbid borderline personality disorder present, especially in combination with self-destructive parental behaviours.

It is unfortunately unsurprising that Michael and Jessie ended up parting ways given the very real challenge that treating NPD presents. However, if Michael's diagnosis had been made earlier, there is a chance that his interpersonally destructive behaviour could have been mitigated. In general, early interventions targeting parenting behaviours and interpersonal interactions are recommended in order to buffer the effects of the problematic behaviours that those with NPD tend to exhibit towards those closest to them.

Take-Home Messages

1. Narcissistic personality disorder is a difficult clinical entity which can present in a variety of ways.
2. No specific treatment recommendations exist for this condition, and it can occur commonly with other personality disorders.

3. It is recommended that a proper assessment of interpersonal relationships as well as the overall functioning of the individual be conducted.
4. When diagnosed early enough, intervention is recommended with regard to parenting aspects of narcissistic personality disorder as this particular personality disorder has been found to have negative impacts on the offspring.
5. Some types of parenting practices such as harsh punishment and lack of affection and nurturing are associated with a high risk for offspring personality disorders that can continue into adulthood.
6. Both problematic paternal and maternal behaviours are associated with elevated risk for offspring personality disorders.
7. Interventions should target improved parental communication and decreased aversive parenting behaviours towards children.
8. It may not always be possible to engage those with personality disorders fully in treatment. However, an approach that involves empathy and focusing on specific types of treatment goals would be helpful to the patient in developing therapeutic alliance.

References

1. Carroll L. A comparative study of narcissism, gender, and sex-role orientation among bodybuilders, athletes, and psychology students. Psychol Rep. 1989;64(3):999–1006.
2. Cramer P. Young adult narcissism: a 20 year longitudinal study of the contribution of parenting styles, preschool precursors of narcissism, and denial. J Res Pers. 2011;45(1):19–28.
3. Cohen O. Parental narcissism and the disengagement of the non-custodial father after divorce. Clin Soc Work J. 1998;26(2):195–215.
4. Dhawan N, Kunik ME, Oldham J, et al. Prevalence and treatment of narcissistic personality disorder in the community: a systematic review. Compr Psychiatry. 2010;51(4):333–9.
5. Elkind D. Instrumental narcissism in parents. Bull Menn Clin. 1991;55(3):299.

6. Elman W, McKelvie S. Narcissism in football players: stereotype or reality. Athl Insight. 2003;5(1):38–46.
7. Grijalva E, Newman DA, Tay L, et al. Gender differences in narcissism: a meta-analytic review. Psychol Bull. 2015;141(2):261.
8. Holtzman NS, Vazire S, Mehl MR. Sounds like a narcissist: behavioral manifestations of narcissism in everyday life. J Res Pers. 2010;44(4):478–84.
9. Johnson JG, Cohen P, Kasen S, et al. Associations of parental personality disorders and axis I disorders with childrearing behavior. Psychiatry. 2006;69(4):336–50.
10. Kraus G, Reynolds DJ. The "ABC's" of the cluster B's: identifying, understanding, and treating cluster B personality disorders. Clin Psychol Rev. 2001;21(3):345–73.
11. Luchner AF, Houston JM, Walker C, et al. Exploring the relationship between two forms of narcissism and competitiveness. Pers Individ Dif. 2011;51(6):779–82.
12. McNeal S. A character in search of character: narcissistic personality disorder and ego state therapy. Am J Clin Hypn. 2003;45(3):233–43.
13. Nadav M, Ephratt M, Rabin S, et al. Names and narcissism: a clinical perspective on how parents choose names for their newborn. Names. 2011;59(2):90–103.
14. Perry JC, Presniak MD, Olson TR. Defense mechanisms in schizotypal, borderline, antisocial, and narcissistic personality disorders. Psychiatry. 2013;76(1):32–52.
15. Philipson I. Gender and narcissism. Psychol Women Q. 1985;9(2):213–28.
16. Porcerelli JH, Sandler BA. Narcissism and empathy in steroid users. Am J Psychiatry. 1995;152(11):1672–4.
17. Rappoport A. Co-narcissism: how we accommodate to narcissistic parents. Therapist. 2005;1:1–8.
18. Thomaes S, Bushman BJ, De Castro BO, et al. What makes narcissists bloom? A framework for research on the etiology and development of narcissism. Dev Psychopathol. 2009;21(4):1233–47.
19. Turner RM. Borderline, narcissistic, and histrionic personality disorders. Handbook of prescriptive treatments for adults. Springer US; 1994. p. 393–420.
20. Twenge JM, Foster JD. Birth cohort increases in narcissistic personality traits among American college students, 1982–2009. Soc Psychol Person Sci 2010;1(1):99–106, 2010 Grant, Bridget F., Ph.D., Ph.D.· Rise B. Goldstein, Ph.D., M.P.H., S. Patricia Chou, Ph.D., Boi Huang, M.D., Ph.D., Frederick S. Stinson, Ph.D.,

Deborah A. Dawson, Ph.D., Tulshi D. Saha, Ph.D., Sharon M. Smith, Ph.D., Atilla J. Pulay, M.D, Roger P. Pickering, M.S., W. June Ruan, M.A., and Wilson M. Compton, M.D., M.P.E.. Sociodemographic and psychopathologic predictors of first incidence of DSM-IV substance use, mood and anxiety disorders: results from the wave 2 national epidemiologic survey on alcohol and related conditions.

21. Trull TJ, Jahng S, Tomko RL, Wood PK, Sher KJ, University of Missouri and Midwest Alcoholism Research Center. Revised NESARC personality disorder diagnoses: gender, prevalence and comorbidity with substance dependence disorders 2010.

22. Stinson FS, Dawson DA, Goldstein RB, Chou SP, Huang B, Smith SM, Ruan WJ, Pulay AJ, Saha TD, Pickering RP, Grant BF. Prevalence, correlates, disability and comorbidity of DSM-IV narcissistic personality disorder: results from the wave 2 national epidemiologic survey on alcohol and related conditions 2008.

23. Tritt SM, Ryder AG, Ring AJ, Pincus AL. Pathological narcissism and the depressive temperament 2009.

Index

© Springer International Publishing AG 2018   189
S.K. Misri, *Paternal Postnatal Psychiatric Illnesses*,
https://doi.org/10.1007/978-3-319-68249-5

Printed in the United States
By Bookmasters